CLINICAL EXAM

passing your
medical finals

WITHDRAWN

CLINICAL EXAMINATION

passing your medical finals

Wai-Ching Leung

MRCP (UK), MRCGP, MRCPsych, DCH, DRCOG, DO, PGCE

*Senior Registrar in Public Health, Northern and Yorkshire Regional
Health Authority, Newcastle-upon-Tyne*

A member of the Hodder Headline Group
LONDON • SYDNEY • AUCKLAND
Copublished in the USA by Oxford University Press, Inc., New York

6/11/96
M

First published in Great Britain in 1996 by
Arnold, a member of the Hodder Headline Group,
338 Euston Road, London NW1 3BH

Co-published in the United States of America by
Oxford University Press, Inc.,
198 Madison Avenue, New York, NY 10016
Oxford is a registered trademark of Oxford University Press

Whilst the advice and information in this book is believed to be true and
accurate at the date of going to press, neither the author nor the publisher
can accept any legal responsibility or liability for any errors or omissions
that may be made.

British Library Cataloguing-in-Publication Data
A catalogue record for this book is available from the British Library

Library of Congress Cataloging-in-Publication Data
A catalog record for this book is available from the Library of Congress

ISBN 0 340 66192 5

Typeset in 11/12 Garamond 3 by Paul Bennett, Tonbridge
Printed and bound in Great Britain by J.W. Arrowsmith Ltd, Bristol

Contents

Foreword		vii
Preface		ix

1 Hints for Preparation
1

Hints for preparation for finals 1
Hints for preparation for continuous assessment 5
Hints for preparation for clinical exams 6

2 General Medicine
11

General advice for long cases 11
Cardiovascular system 18
Diabetes 24
Respiratory system 25
Presentation of short cases 31
The abdomen – alimentary and genitourinary systems 31
Neurological system 42
Diseases of joints 51
Examples of association of skin lesions with systemic disease 54
Example of a general medicine long case 54

3 General Surgery
58

General advice for long cases 58
Short cases 60
Example of a general surgery long case 74

4 Paediatrics
78

General advice for long cases 78
List of equipment 84
Cardiovascular system 85
Respiratory system 89
Abdomen 93
Neurology 95
Development assessment 99
Squints 104
Common syndromes seen in exams 106
Example of a paediatric long case 107

5 Obstetrics **112**
General advice for long cases 112
Routine antenatal investigations 118
Anaemia in pregnancy 119
Rhesus incompatibility 120
Pregnancy-induced hypertension (pre-eclampsia) 120
Antepartum haemorrhage 121
Established diabetes and pregnancy 123
Labour 123
Example of an obstetrics long case 126

6 Gynaecology **129**
General advice for long cases 129
Abortion 133
Abnormal uterine bleeding 135
Amenorrhoea 137
Dysmenorrhoea 137
Vaginal discharge 138
Infertility 139
Gynaecological cancers 140
Contraception 141
Genital (uterine) prolapse 143
Example of a gynaecological long case 144

7 Psychiatry **147**
General advice for long cases 147
Organic causes of psychiatric disorders – delirium 155
Diagnosis of schizophrenia 156
Findings from history and on examination 157
Comparison of findings in mania/hypomania and depression 157
Assessing risk of suicide 157
Neurotic disorders 161
Dementia 162
Alcohol abuse 164
Example of a psychiatric long case 166

8 General Practice **171**
What general practice can offer to students 171
History taking, examination and presentation 172
Future assessment of undergraduates in general practice 175

Index **176**

Foreword

The transition from medical student to doctor is one of enormous importance, not just for the individual making it, but for the health service of the country whose workforce the new entrant is joining and for patients both present and future. Traditionally, entry to the medical profession has only taken place after a rigorous process of assessment and examination based on an educational programme in an approved institution.

Whilst fashions in methods of assessment in education and training have changed over time and vary from place to place, standards must of necessity remain high. Many schools of medicine include a formal clinical examination of patients as an important part of the process of student assessment. This format has the capacity to instil great trepidation in students. An unfamiliar situation far removed from the relative comfort of the written examination paper, having to be observed, having little time to reflect on the matters at hand, the possibility of making a wrong response which could be construed as having serious clinical consequences and the need to be sensitive to the patient's needs and wishes all add to the stress and anxiety.

Dr Leung's book provides a comprehensive and valuable guide to prepare students for this important format of assessment. It deserves to take its place amongst the small number of apprenticeship texts which successive generations of students keep close to their sides.

Professor Liam Donaldson
Professor of Applied Epidemiology
University of Newcastle upon Tyne
United Kingdom

May 1996

Preface

The assessment of patients through history taking and clinical examination, and the subsequent presentation of their cases, is an important skill for the student to learn. A medical student will be required to exercise this skill in teaching ward rounds, in clinical meeting and clinico-pathological conferences, in continuous assessment schemes and in the finals exam.

The clinical component has always been the most important part of the finals exam, and quite rightly so. In this, candidates demonstrate to the examiner their competence in clinical skills and whether they are safe to be qualified. Most students who fail do so because of inadequate performance in this part of their exam. Most candidates feel least confident and most nervous in this aspect of finals, as hours of book work will not necessarily see them through this.

Another problem is that the approaches to cases in different specialities (general medicine, surgery, paediatrics, obstetrics, gynaecology and psychiatry) are different. This makes it even more difficult for the candidates to revise, as they need to consult different sections of different textbooks. Indeed, there is a danger that candidates may concentrate on some specialities to the total exclusion of others, with the result of total panic when one is facing in finals cases from specialities that one has not prepared. I knew of one colleague some years ago who spent hours rehearsing general medicine cases for his medical finals clinicals, but was at a loss when then presented with psychiatric cases.

In the publication *Tomorrow's Doctors*, the General Medical Council (December 1993) recommended that the 'Basic clinical method' – including the ability to (a) obtain and record a comprehensive history; (b) perform a complete physical examination, and assess the mental state; (c) interpret the findings obtained from the history and the physical examination; and (d) reach a provisional assessment of patients' problems and formulate with them plans for investigation and management – was designated as one of the two skills objectives in the future 'core curriculum'. It is clear, therefore, that this skill will in the future continue to be regarded as a very important part of the medical curriculum.

Many clinical schools assess their students by a combination of continuous assessment and finals exam, and there is a trend towards the continuous assessment component occupying a larger proportion of the total assessment. While this trend may help students with 'examination nerves', it places a heavier burden on students to 'find their feet' in new firms as quickly as possible, and to be able to give a reliable, relevant and concise history and examination of their patients on the ward rounds in order to give a good impression. Appreciation of how to present cases in different specialities becomes even more important as there is a danger that students present their cases in the same style as for their previous firm (e.g. psychiatric cases in the same style a general medicine ones) which would not be appropriate. The General Medical Council report recommends that students should spend more time in general practice, as history taking and physical examination in this area is quite different from that in hospital specialities.

This book attempts to give students general hints on different approaches in different specialities to obtain a reliable, relevant and concise history and examination from their patients and present them either in finals or in their continuous assessment clinical attachments in an effective manner. It concentrates on the main undergraduate specialities in which students are expected to present cases. Postgraduate specialities, such as ophthalmology, ENT and orthopaedics, are deliberately omitted, as students would not be expected to present such patients in detail. This book will be useful for both long and short cases in the final exam and for students who join a firm in a new speciality. It also summarizes useful basic information about different cases that are especially likely to come up in the long cases, and about the clinical signs that students may be expected to demonstrate in the short cases of finals or in ward rounds of different specialities. It is not, of course, intended to be comprehensive.

1
Hints for Preparation

Hints for preparation for finals

If the assessment by your clinical school is by finals exam, you have the advantage that the assessment is carried out by examiners who do not know you, and hence they are more likely to be more objective. You may be relieved that you do not have the continuous psychological pressure of having to 'please' your consultants and may feel free to ask questions without fear of showing your ignorance and hence jeopardizing your assessment results. The finals exam also provides you with good practice for your postgraduate exams a few years after you qualify, which are compulsory if you wish to enter into any hospital speciality and strongly recommended if you wish to enter general practice.

However, being assessed by a final exam means that you need to be well prepared for almost all specialities at the end of your course (some medical schools hold exams in some subjects, pathology and obstetrics and gynaecology in particular, in the year before the main finals exam), and you need to retain your proficiency in all specialities until the end of the course.

Although the finals exam may seem formidable, the chance of your passing it is very high (in excess of 95%). You are almost guaranteed to succeed if you have worked reasonably conscientiously throughout your course, turned up reasonably regularly for your clinical attachments and adhered to a sound revision schedule.

The finals exams themselves differ between clinical schools but are likely to consist of:

- pharmacology and therapeutics;
- pathology;
- obstetrics and gynaecology;
- general medicine (including public health), paediatrics and psychiatry may be examined by separate papers;
- general surgery (including ENT, ophthalmology and orthopaedics).

Pathology is usually examined by multiple choice questions (MCQ), short answers or essay questions, a practical and a viva. Pharmacology and therapeutics is usually examined by MCQs, short answer or essay questions and a viva. The clinical subjects are examined by a combination of MCQs, short answer or essay questions, a clinical examination and a viva.

Although different methods of preparation may suit different students, the following general advice may be given.

DURING THE CLINICAL COURSE

There are often family and social pressures around you, leaving you to doubt whether you have worked sufficiently to pass the finals exam. There are always a few who appear to 'know everything' in ward rounds, a few who are found in the library every moment, which may make you anxious about your own performance. However, it is essential to have a balanced view of the medical course and be sceptical about sacrificing other interests and social life at this early stage of a medical career, bearing in mind that steady and systematic work will nearly guarantee success in finals and that exams and continuous education continue for many years to come after you qualify.

Lectures and seminars

It is well known that some lecturers and their lectures are excellent while some are next to useless. Also, some students learn a great deal by attending lectures and making notes, while others learn by reading textbooks themselves. However, it is generally advisable to go to at least the first few lectures in each series rather than deciding by word of mouth from your fellow students that they are not for you. Even if you do decide that you learn better by studying textbooks on your own, it is important to ask your fellow students what topics were taught in the lectures and browse through the notes they made and the handouts that were given. In this way, you have some idea of the topics and level of understanding required in the exam.

Seminars and supervisions are generally indispensable. The number of students is less, you have the opportunity to ask the questions you want to and it also helps you to develop the skills of presenting patients, listening to your fellow students' presentations and discussing the management of the patients. This skill is, of course, vital in your finals exam. You will also receive some informal feedback on how you are progressing.

Notes and textbooks

Some students benefit from making copious notes both during and outside lectures, while others depend exclusively on good textbooks.

This is a matter of personal preference and, in general, making notes is only useful if they are legible and well organized. Otherwise, you may be better off choosing a good manageable textbook at the beginning of the study of each speciality and highlighting the points you need to revise in the future.

It is more economical, and better for your learning, to buy a reasonably concise textbook and know it well rather than choose an over-ambitious textbook and get baffled and discouraged by it. In general, studying a good concise textbook in detail will give you a firm basis for the subject and is more likely to allow you to see the wood from the trees, a skill that is vital in the finals exam. Indeed, persistently mentioning rare before common causes in the finals exam is an important reason for failure. You can always use as a reference a more detailed library textbook to elaborate on topics in which you are interested. As a rule of thumb, a medium-sized, good textbook of less than 300 pages is sufficient for any one speciality.

Clinical attachments

It cannot be stressed enough that regular attendance and practice in obtaining history and performing physical examinations on patients is the most important preparation for the finals exam; this cannot be substituted for by the study of textbooks. Make use of opportunities to present your cases in ward rounds and to consultants or junior doctors, both in inpatient and outpatient settings.

REVISION FOR FINALS

It is advisable to start revising about 6 months before your finals. Depending on the organization of your clinical course, you are most likely to be in your senior medical or surgical firm. A revision schedule of 2 hours revision an evening on weekdays, and probably 5 hours revision at weekends, is probably realistic and sufficient if the revision time is used efficiently. It is important that you make a list of topics you are going to revise, taking into account the topics covered by the course lectures. It is wise to start off with specialities that you completed a while previously.

It is important to take breaks and revise in periods of no more than 1 hour. It is difficult to concentrate effectively for a longer time, and attempts to revise for longer periods are likely to yield little progress.

Revision for finals should consist of the following:

- Revise from your notes and/or your chosen textbooks. You should have decided during your course whether you are going to make notes or are going to use a textbook that you highlight and make marginal notes in. It is important that you stick to your choice during your revision. Make a list of topics that you may want to look up in more detailed reference books when you are next in the library. If you find these books useful, make a note in your textbook of the page number of the reference book or, alternatively, write brief notes in your file and/or keep a photocopy of the reference book entry in your file.

- Practise your MCQ techniques by doing MCQs from revision books on the market or MCQs given to you during your course. You can either attempt the MCQs before revising the topic to work out which are your weak topics or attempt the MCQs after revising the appropriate topics. To start off with, do not attempt more than half a MCQ test a night, and try to work out from your textbook or revision notes the answers that you got wrong. When it is near to your exam, try to familiarize yourself with the format of the exam by completing an MCQ under exam conditions.

- It is important not to forget many 'smaller topics', for example, 'postgraduate' specialities (e.g. ophthalmology, ENT and orthopaedics) and other topics, such as public health medicine, law and ethics, which may feature in some of the MCQs. Find out in advance which of the topics are on the syllabus.

- After you revise the appropriate topics, try to answer the short questions and outline your answers to the essay questions. Check your answers from your textbook and discuss your approach to the essay questions with your supervisor or fellow students.

- Highlight the points you need to revise further in different colours.

- If possible, form a study group with your fellow students and plan the topics you are going to revise in each session. Studying in groups and discussions with your fellow students are often more effective than working on your own.

- Grasp every chance to see patients under exam conditions and present patients to other doctors. Ward rounds, attending new outpatients and shadowing a registrar on call provide good opportunities. You must be aware of the different emphasis in history taking and examination in different specialities. Try to organize with your supervisor chances to see and present patients in specialities that you completed some time ago.

THE WEEK BEFORE YOUR FINALS

It is important that you do not stay up late at night studying, as this is unlikely to be effective at this stage. Having a reasonable social life and occasionally engaging in other interests will help you to think and answer questions with good common sense in the exam, which is more important than knowing minute details.

At this stage, you should not attempt to study from long, detailed textbooks or textbooks that you have not used before, as their different approaches are more likely to confuse you than help you.

Your revision should take account of the following:

- Make sure that you know the format of your exam well, and practise old question papers and/or papers from published revision books. Revise your weak topics, as shown by the practice tests.
- Read through your highlighted notes/textbooks and try to have a good knowledge of the symptoms, signs and management of the common disorders than knowledge of rare syndromes.
- Plan very carefully how you are going to present your long and short cases in you clinical exam in each speciality. Write them down in note form.
- Practise presenting long cases and being examined in short cases by asking registrars in your firm to give you a mock clinical exam.

Hints for preparation for continuous assessment

The advantages of this method of assessment are that you need to revise for one speciality at a time and that there are more opportunities to resit the assessment without delaying your date of qualification by 6 months should you be unsuccessful in your first attempt. You will also be assessed, at least partly, by the consultants in your firm, so 'nerves' should not be a cause for failure.

The disadvantage is, however, that you are continually being observed and assessed, and there is continuous pressure on you to give a 'good impression' from the first day you are on the firm. It is probably true to say that your consultants are more likely than are external examiners to be influenced by subjective factors, such as your gender, ethnic origin, social class and personality, although they should have been made aware of the dangers of being influenced by such factors.

It is most important that you behave professionally during your clinical attachment. This includes being reliable (turning up for every session you can and informing your consultant in advance if you will be absent), punctual, courteous and considerate to the patients, and trying to get on well with other staff, such as nursing staff and social workers. Indeed, an impression of being late all the time and an inability to get on with patients and staff will have a disastrous effect on your assessment that cannot be compensated for by accurate, concise, articulate presentation and outstanding knowledge.

You should find out the 'rule' of your firm on your first day, either from other students, the junior doctors or your consultants. Find out who usually presents cases in the ward rounds and how patients are shared between the students. You should know the history and progress of the patients allocated to you and always be prepared to present your patients if required. Remember that, even if the junior doctors usually present the cases, they may be called away during the ward round and you may be unexpectedly asked to present the cases. Try to get a feel for how much detail is expected when presenting your cases (as either too much or too little detail may give a bad impression), and the aspects that the consultants regard as particularly important in the ward round. Also try to find out the time of the teaching sessions and which patients you are expected to have seen beforehand. You should be familiar with the history taking, physical examination and presentation technique appropriate to the specialty.

As far as theoretical considerations are concerned, the advice given in 'Hints for preparation for finals' above also applies here. You must know how you will be assessed on your theoretical knowledge, which may be by MCQs or by short answer/essay questions. You should read up about the conditions that you saw clinically, as you are more likely then to understand and remember them.

Unlike in assessment by finals exam, you will be assessed on your theoretical knowledge shortly after you complete your relevant clinical attachments. Hence, you need to plan your revision half way into your clinical attachment, and you should have selected and bought your chosen textbook when you started your clinical attachment.

Hints for preparation for clinical exams

The keys to preparation for clinicals are given below:

- *Know what features in the history and examination are important to elicit for each specialty.* An obvious example is that 'last menstrual period' and 'contraceptive history' are important in obstetrics and gynaecology, but may not be important in other specialities. The important features must be so well known that you develop a routine and know what to ask for automatically without any conscious effort to recall and without missing any important information.
- *Being able to present the history and examination smoothly and flexibly, depending on how much detail is required by the examiners/consultants.*

This can only be achieved if a set of routines are understood and practised repeatedly. An example is to know the routine of examining and presenting the examination findings for the abdomen in an obstetrics case of 'appearance, fundal height, lie, presentation, engagement, back of fetus and fetal heart'. Without having learnt and practised this routine, it is unlikely that the candidate would be able to present the findings logically and efficiently.

- *Gain sufficient practice in interviewing patients and presenting cases.* Knowing the 'lists' required for each specialty is only the first step. This must be practised again and again by interviewing and examining patients and presenting them in front of others (preferably consultants or junior doctors).

GENERAL HINTS IN THE FINAL CLINICAL EXAM

Irrespective of the particular specialty, the following points are important when taking a clinical exam.

- You must find out in advance exactly how much time you are allowed to see the patient, to gather your thoughts, to present your case, to see the patient with the examiners and for the examiners to question you afterwards. You should also find out which specialities may be used in the examination. For example, in some clinical schools, psychiatric, paediatric or general medicine cases may appear in a medical long case, and obstetrics, gynaecology or family planning patients may appear in an obstetrics and gynaecology exam.
- You should also avoid staying up late or reading about obscure topics the previous night. If you wish to revise, remind yourself of the important points of the history and examination in those particular specialities, and perhaps quickly browse through the symptoms, signs, investigations and management of their *common* conditions. You should always go to bed early the previous night.
- On the day of the exam, you should dress formally and conservatively. This has always been the tradition, and doing something different from others may make you more anxious and it also creates a poor impression. You should aim to arrive at your exam centre in good time, allowing for unforeseen circumstances.
- If possible, try to bring your own equipment, which you are used to. You should have your stethoscope and probably your own ophthalmoscope. Having equipment you are familiar with will certainly help you a great deal in your physical examination.

LONG CASES

Interviewing the patient

Be very sceptical about any diagnosis for the patient that you may have heard from other candidates. They may be talking about another patient – or they may be wrong! In any case, you will need to explain your reasoning in reaching your conclusions.

Be courteous to the patient, introduce yourself and explain that you are in an exam and that you need to ask several questions and perform a physical examination in a short time. Informing them that you are a student prevents them from asking you questions about their treatment. Getting the patient on your side is a great help, and he or she may even tell you the diagnosis.

Before you start, to take the history, write in bold the headings in the order you are used to on the papers provided, leaving plenty of space to write your notes. In this way, it will remind you of the important features to enquire of in the history, and if you have to deviate from the routine, you can still present your findings from your notes in the usual way.

You must have a rough guide for the time you allocate to history taking, physical examination and thinking about the case, although the exact duration you spend on each aspect depends on the particular case. Watch the time carefully, covering the important features first (e.g. history of presenting complaint or relevant past history), and then the physical examination of the relevant system, leaving other less important details (e.g. routine systemic enquiries and neurological examination in a patient with gastrointestinal complaints) to the end.

Always ask the patient the following questions:

- What did the other doctors say the matter was? (Most patients will tell you. If the patient replies, 'That's for you to find out' take it graciously!)
- What drug treatment are you on at present?
- What other treatment (e.g. physiotherapy or occupational therapy) are you having at present?
- Are there any other questions you think I should have asked you?

Always test the urine if it is provided.

Allow yourself 5–10 minutes to make a list of the differential diagnoses and treatment plan. Try also to prepare a succinct summary of your presentation, which you will need either at the end of your presentation or at the beginning if the examiners ask for it. Write it down clearly. For example:

Mrs X is a 29-year-old primigravida now 38 weeks into her pregnancy, with a long history of insulin-dependent diabetes, who has presented with a 5-day history of symptoms of pre-eclampsia – raised blood pressure, oedema and proteinuria – and has been admitted for bed rest and observation.

Interview with the examiners

In your presentation, you must strike a balance between giving a comprehensive presentation and being long-winded. You should be constantly aware of the examiners' non-verbal communication. In general, state all the positive points and relevant negative points in the history and examination, but not a list of irrelevant negatives. For example, the statement, 'There was no anaemia, no cyanosis, no clubbing and no lymphadenopathy' as a routine is totally unnecessary.

Avoid reading from the notes throughout the presentation. Look at the examiners from time to time, and try to vary the tone of your voice to make your presentation interesting.

You should conclude your presentation with the concise summary that you prepared beforehand. You will then be asked to demonstrate certain features in the history or, more commonly, demonstrate the patient's positive physical sign(s) in front of the examiners. You should:

- Show courtesy and consideration to the patient, especially if the patient needs to be undressed for the examination.
- Show thoroughness in the examination. Remember that you should examine the patient as if you have not examined him or her before. If asked to examine the abdomen, you must go through the procedure of 'observation, light palpation, deep palpation, percussion and auscultation', even if you know from your previous examination that there is nothing positive on observation. Try to give a running commentary as you go along. For example, when observing the abdomen, say to the examiner, 'The abdomen is not visibly distended, and there is no peristalsis seen. There is a scar in the right iliac fossa, which appears to be an appendicectomy scar.'

After examining the patient, help the patient to dress and thank him or her before leaving.

The examiners will then take you to another room to ask you about the differential diagnosis and management. In the discussion of the differential diagnosis, give the most common and likely diagnosis first and leave the uncommon causes until later. It is much more important to give all the common causes than to give numerous, obscure, rarer ones. Likewise, in the management, think of simple measures first (e.g. analgesia or bed rest) and leave the experimental high-powered treatment until the end.

SHORT CASES

The short cases are perhaps the most important and the most anxiety-provoking part of the examination. You are led by two examiners to see as many cases as possible in the time allotted. In each case, you are asked to examine a particular system (cardiovascular, respiratory, etc.).

Listen very carefully to what the examiner asks you. For example, if the instruction is, 'Examine the cardiovascular system', then you should quickly but efficiently look for signs of cyanosis, oedema and raised jugular venous pressure (JVP) and examine the peripheral pulses for rate, rhythm and volume, etc. If the instruction is, 'Listen to the heart', you should do as you are told, and avoid annoying the examiners by going through the above list. If the instruction is, 'Examine the heart', you should probably mention quickly that you would like to do all the above, and start with looking for the apex beat and palpating for thrills and heave, before listening to the heart.

Give a running commentary of what you are doing. This saves time at the end to present your findings and prevents you forgetting what you have found! Also, if you are on the wrong track, kind examiners may point this out to you.

Be thorough and methodical. For example, in examining the respiratory system, you should first look for cyanosis and clubbing, then observe the chest for deformities, scars, respiratory rate, Harrison's sulcus, intercostal and subcostal recession, etc., then palpate for vocal fremitus, then perform percussion methodically and end with auscultation of the chest. You should have developed a routine for examining each individual system.

Give the differential diagnosis after your presentation of your findings. Start with the most common or most likely first. If you might be able to distinguish between differential diagnoses by examining another system, say so.

See as many short cases as possible in the given time. Hence, your examination, while thorough, needs to be quick and efficient. If the examiners ask you to focus on a particular point (e.g. auscultation) while you are still observing, do as you are told. This may mean that they are satisfied that you would be thorough but that, in the interests of time, they want to see what else you would find.

Be courteous and professional.

2
General Medicine

General advice for long cases

Students are probably more confident about history taking, physical examination and presentation in general medicine than in other specialities, as the initial teaching on basic clinical skills often commences in a general medical firm and the average student spends more time on general medical than on most other firms.

In general medicine, important information may occur under *any* heading in the history or in examination of any system. Therefore, it is important, when you are taking the history of the present complaint(s), to think of possible diagnoses so that important relevant questions can be tackled in the rest of the history and examination. Except in the very early stages of your clinical training, asking a huge list of rote-learnt, predetermined questions (e.g. asking about tuberculosis, jaundice or rheumatic fever in the past medical history) is quite pointless: ask only what appears relevant.

HISTORY (25 minutes)

Personal details

Name: Sex:
Age/d.o.b.:   Occupation:

Presenting complaint(s)

List the complaints briefly, using the patient's own words if possible (e.g. 'feeling faint', 'indigestion').

History of presenting complaint(s)

It is especially important to record exactly when symptoms start, how they progress and what treatment (including self-medication) is used and when.

For example:

6/12 [6 months] ago – Experienced acid in the mouth especially when lying down. No treatment taken.

3/12 ago – Started having pain in the upper abdomen, sharp, lasting for 2–4 hours each time. Needed to lie down when this occurred. Improved with drinking milk, got worse when hungry. Initially occurred only once every week, then progressed to once a day 6 weeks ago. Saw GP, given Asilone liquid 10 ml tds, partial relief.

4/7 [4 days] ago – Noted to be passing black stools. Did not seek help.

1/7 ago – Collapsed while at work and was brought to hospital. Found to have Hb of 5 g/dL. Given 4 units of blood yesterday.

When you are told a symptom, listen to the patient's story. At the end, make sure you know the answers to the questions in Box 2.1 or clarify points with the patient. (Not all of the these questions are, of course, necessarily appropriate.)

Box 2.1. Questions that may be asked for any symptoms

1. Onset (When did it start?)
2. Progression (Has it got better, worse or been unchanged since it started?)
3. Frequency (How often does it come on?)
4. Duration (How often does it last for each time?)
5. Severity (How bad is it? What do you do when you have it?)
6. Character (What is it like?)
7. Relieving factors (What makes it better?)
8. Aggravating factors (What makes it worse?)
9. Associated symptoms (What other symptoms do you have with it?)

For example, for a patient complaining of headache, you may obtain the history as:

The headache is mostly frontal and occipital; it started 6 months ago as a dull ache, and occurred once a week. Since then, it has become more frequent, occurring daily in the last month, and the pain has become sharper and associated with vomiting and nausea; he sees flashing lights in front of both eyes. When it occurs, he has to stay in bed in a dark room, usually for 4–8 hours. He has noticed that eating cheese occasionally makes it worse, but taking a paracetamol tablet makes it less severe.

The cause of the headache becomes more apparent with these enquiries.

Past medical history

The main items to elicit, in strict chronological order, are shown in Box 2.2.

Box 2.2. Past medical history

1. history that may contribute to the presenting complaint(s)
2. chronic conditions
3. conditions that may recur (e.g. peptic ulcer), relapse (e.g. multiple sclerosis) or give rise to complications. Again, pay particular attention to whether the presenting complaints may be complications of past illnesses (e.g. rheumatic fever when valvular heart disease is suspected)
4. any major surgical operations and the primary diagnosis
5. foreign travel (especially recent, and any any immunization or prophylactic treatment taken)

You need not include childhood infections (unless relevant, such as chickenpox in suspected herpes zoster and measles in undiagnosed neurological conditions.) Do not include common colds, viral infections, etc.

For example, for a patient presenting with an unexplained left leg paralysis:

1980 – Admitted to Allcure Hospital for 3 days with epigastric pain, duodenal ulcer diagnosed endoscopically, treated with 6/52 [6 weeks] course of cimetidine.

1982 – Admitted to Tophernia Hospital for elective repair of right indirect inguinal hernia.

1985 – Sudden loss of eyesight for 2 weeks, seen by ophthalmologist in Alleye Hospital, treated with steroids (?dose), diagnosed 'optic nerve inflammation'. Patient remembered visual field examination being performed and was warned that there was a chance of relapse.

1986 – Mild hypertension noted by GP, given bendrofluazide 5 mg daily. Under control since.

1988 – Sudden loss of power right arm, tingling sensation left arm. Admitted to local psychiatric hospital, diagnosed ?hysteria, symptoms disappeared after 2 weeks with no treatment.

1991 – Diagnosed irritable bowel syndrome, given Fybogel, symptoms settled after 6 months.

Details of the history from 1985 and 1988 are the most relevant and their investigation should be given priority if time is about to run out.

Drug history

All drugs taken, whether prescribed or not, should be recorded, along with their dosage and frequency and how long they have been taken for.

For example:

Cimetidine 400mg bd (in last year)
Maxolon 10mg tds (in last 4 weeks)
Chlorpromazine 25mg tds (in last 2 weeks)
Paracetamol 1g tds as required

Allergies

Do not just accept patients' accounts of what they are 'allergic' to. Ask, for example, when the relevant drug was taken and what the reaction was (e.g. many patients describe feeling nauseous after taking penicillin as being 'allergic' to it).

Family history

It is generally easier to draw a traditional 'pedigree chart':

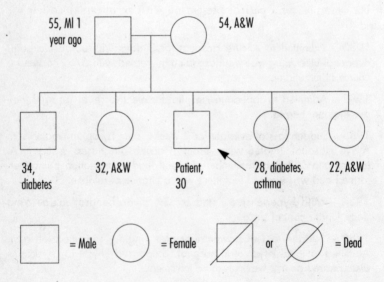

2.1 Example of a pedigree chart

The two reasons for taking family history are that:

1. Some diseases are hereditary, either:
   (a) *chromosomally*, for example, balanced translocation of Down's syndrome;
   (b) *by single gene transmission*, for example, as an autosomal dominant such as Marfan's syndrome, autosomal recessive such as Wilson's disease, sex-linked recessive such as haemophilia or sex-linked dominant such as vitamin D-resistant rickets;
   (c) *polygenic*, for example, diabetes.
2. Some diseases (e.g. cancer) are not genetic, but patients may worry (probably unnecessarily) that they have the same disease as other members of the family. Knowledge of family history will help the clinician to reassure the patient.

You should aim to take into account only serious or genetic illness in the family; you must be selective.

Social history

Smoking and alcohol
With increasing emphasis on preventive medicine in the Health of the Nation strategy, examiners are likely in the future to place more emphasis on this part of the history. Patients may be evasive about this aspect of their lifestyle. Try to probe gently. For alcohol, convert the intake into units if possible. Use the CAGE questionnaire if necessary (*see* section on 'Alcohol abuse' in Chapter 7).

Occupation
Enquire about both present and past occupations.

- Occupation-related disease (e.g. asbestos exposure predisposing to mesothelioma or a pub owner being more likely to have an alcohol problem).
- A decline in occupational level may be associated with physical (or mental) disabilities.
- Unemployment may be associated with increasing physical and mental illness.

Home and social situation

- Living accommodation – number of rooms, which floor (if the patient has reduced mobility).
- Who is living with the patient? How is he or she getting on with them?
- Financial situation, and social support he or she is receiving (e.g. meals on wheel, home help).

Interests
Make a note of the patient's interests and hobbies.

Systemic enquiries

Students are often told to go through a whole checklist of symptoms to ensure that there are no unsuspected diseases or symptoms that are missed. This may be useful in the first 3 or 4 weeks of one's clinical training, when trying to become familiarized with the symptoms of each system.

However, in the long run this approach causes too many problems, especially in an exam. First, patients often get so frustrated with such an exhaustive list that they lose their concentration or even refuse to co-operate. Second, many patients reply positively to many of these symptoms, with no particular significance. Third, you simply have not got the time in the finals exam to go through all the questions.

What I would suggest is that you go through the cardinal symptoms of the system relevant to the presenting complaint(s). For example, if the presenting complaint is shortness of breath, go through the cardinal symptoms of both cardiovascular and respiratory systems (which you probably have anyway in the history of presenting complaints). Leave the rest until the end (if you still have the time) or until during the physical examination, when you can ask the patient the relevant questions while examining the particular system (e.g. ask about gastrointestinal symptoms when you are examining the abdomen).

The cardinal symptoms of each system are listed in the subsequent sections.

PHYSICAL EXAMINATION (20 minutes)

You must be selective in your examination. If the presenting complaint is chest pain, you must examine the cardiovascular system in detail, but you do not need to go through each cranial nerve.

General

There are so many general features to look for that you must choose those which are relevant to the presenting complaint(s). One often looks for anaemia, cyanosis, lymphadenopathy, jaundice, clubbing and any unusual features on first impression. There is no particular rationale for this, apart from the fact that the findings give a clue to many diseases.

A list of general features to look for in any particular system is given overleaf.

Particular systems

Detailed examination of each particular system is given below.

Urine

If urine is provided, it must be tested whatever the presenting complaint(s)! One can almost always think of a valid reason for doing so.

PRESENTATION

Always prepare a short written summary. The examiner may ask for the summary to start with, but in any case you need to give a summary at the end.

An example of a summary is:

> A 40-year-old divorced businessman who was admitted 3 days ago with acute severe haematemesis of bright red blood. He had a duodenal ulcer 5 years ago demonstrated endoscopically, which was treated with a course of triple antibiotics. He has drunk 60 units of alcohol a week for the past 2 years. Examination revealed the stigmata of liver diseases and signs of portal hypertension.

Then proceed with your differential diagnosis.

It is perhaps also wise to prepare the first sentence of your presentation to give you the necessary confidence. Remember to give details of each *important* symptom, as well as of important negatives. In the past medical, family and social histories, you must be concise yet show that you are looking for relevant points by including relevant negative points. For example, in a case of neurofibromatosis, say, 'There is no family history of neurofibromatosis'. In a case of contact dermatitis, carefully mention negative points in the occupational history.

For systemic enquiries, it is sufficient to say, 'There are no other symptoms in the systemic enquiries except ...'. Similarly, in physical examination of a patient presenting with chest pain, it is sufficient to say, 'Neurological examination was intact'. If the examiner wants to know more, he or she will ask you.

Always prepare a list of differential diagnoses and be ready to give reasons for or against each diagnosis. Also be prepared to comment on management.

Cardiovascular system

HISTORY

History of presenting complaint(s)

Box 2.3. Cardinal symptoms of heart disease

- chest pain
- shortness of breath
- palpitation
- oedema

 Chest pain

Box 2.4. Characteristic pain of angina

- site – retrosternal
- radiation – both (especially left) hands, arm, jaw
- character – 'tight band'
- aggravating factors – exercise, after a meal, cold
- relieving factors – rest, warmth, glyceryl trinitrate (GTN)
- associated features – breathlessness

Box 2.5. Differentiation of pain of myocardial infarction from that of angina

- aggravating factors – not necessarily precipitated by exercise
- relieving factors – not relieved by rest
- severity – more severe

Box 2.6. Differentiation of pain of pericarditis from that of angina

- aggravating factors – inspiration, change of posture
- relieving factors – analgesia, especially non-steroidal anti-inflammatory drugs (NSAIDs)
- character – stabbing pain
- associated sign – pericardial rub

Breathlessness (dyspnoea)

> **Box 2.7. Characteristic features of pulmonary oedema**
>
> - breathlessness on exercise or at rest
> - cough with white, frothy sputum
> - sputum may be slightly blood stained
> - aggravating factor – lying flat (orthopnoea)
> - relieving factor – sitting up
> - associated signs – pale, sweaty, poor perfusion, widespread crepitations

Palpitation

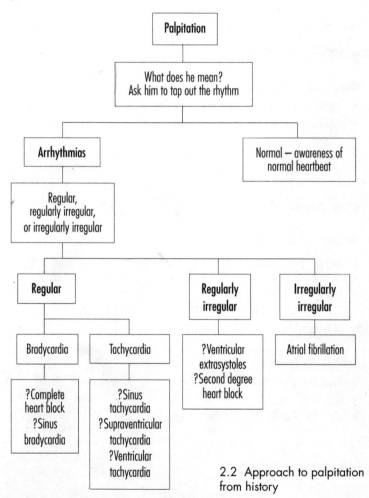

2.2 Approach to palpitation from history

Oedema

Box 2.8. Causes of oedema

- fluid overload:
  - cardiac failure
  - renal disease, e.g. acute glomerulonephritis
- low oncotic pressure – hypoalbuminaemia:
  - nephrotic syndrome: loss of albumin in urine
  - liver disease
  - malnutrition, e.g. kwashiorkor

It is important not to attribute heart failure as a cause of peripheral oedema unless there are other symptoms (e.g. shortness of breath).

Past medical history

Box 2.9. Past medical history

- rheumatic fever
- cardiac or respiratory disease (including hypertension)
- diabetes
- high plasma cholesterol level
- recent viral illness

Family history

Box 2.10. Family history

- angina, myocardial infarction
- diabetes
- high plasma cholesterol level

Social history

Box 2.11. Social history

- smoking
- alcohol intake
- occupation – will the symptoms affect his or her job?

Associated symptoms

- fever (in bacterial endocarditis)
- oliguria or haematuria
- syncope (in arrhythmia)
- abdominal pain (liver congestion)

PHYSICAL EXAMINATION

General

- signs of high cholesterol – corneal arcus, xanthelasma
- malar flush – in mitral disease
- anaemia
- cyanosis
- clubbing
- splinter haemorrhages – under nails and in palate
- fever
- assess thyroid status, palpate thyroid and look for signs of Graves' disease
- optic fundus – for haemorrhages (in endocarditis), hypertensive changes or diabetic changes

Cardiovascular system

- *pulse* – rate, rhythm, character (slow rising in aortic stenosis, collapsing in aortic incompetence). Look for radio-femoral delay if coarctation of the aorta is suspected
- *blood pressure* – specify whether this was taken lying, sitting or standing
- *JVP* – measured from the sternal angle: may be an abnormal waveform ('cannon waves' in complete heart block is the usual abnormality that students are expected to diagnose)
- *oedema* – especially ankle and (for less mobile patients) sacral

Chest

- *inspection* – for visible cardiac impulses and double apex beat
- *palpation:*
  - apex beat: usually 5th intercostal space, mid-clavicular line
  - heave: left or right ventricular hypertrophy
  - thrills: palpable murmurs, at least grade 4/6
- *auscultation:*
  - listen to the whole area of the precordium, especially both sides of the sternal edge, lower left sternal edge and apex

— listen for the first and second heart sounds, splitting of the second heart sound and the presence of any murmurs
— listen for radiations of murmurs to the carotid arteries (for the aortic valve) and under the axilla (for the mitral valve)
— accentuate the mitral valve by lying the patient on the left side; use the bell of the stethoscope for listening to a mitral stenosis murmur
— accentuate the aortic valve by having the patient sit up, lean forwards and hold the breath in expiration. Use the diaphragm of the stethoscope

Location of a heart valve murmur
Note:

• the location of the murmur does not always correspond to the surface markings of heart valves
• murmurs radiate in the direction of blood flow relating to the murmur (*see* Table 2.1):
  — mitral valve: loudest at the apex
  — aortic valve: loudest at the right upper sternal edge
  — tricuspid valve: loudest at the lower left sternal edge
  — pulmonary valve: loudest at the upper left sternal edge

Box 2.12. How to describe a murmur

• maximal site
• sites of radiation
• pitch
• intensity (grade out of 6)
• systolic or diastolic
• which part of systole or diastole (or state how many quarters of systole, for example, it occupies)
• what manoeuvres accentuate it

Box 2.13. How to describe the intensity of a murmur

• grade 1 – just audible in ideal conditions
• grade 2 – quiet
• grade 3 – quite loud, but no thrill
• grade 4 – loud with thrill
• grade 5 – very loud
• grade 6 – audible without stethoscope

Table 2.1. A brief summary of the physical examination of the heart valves

Condition	Pulse/JVP	Blood pressure	Apex beat	Palpation	Auscultation
Mitral stenosis	May have atrial fibrillation	Normal	Tapping (palpable first heart sound)	Heave of left side of sternum (right ventricular hypertrophy)	Loud first heart sound, opening snap, low-pitched, mid-diastolic murmur
Mitral regurgitation	Normal	Normal	Displaced left ventricular dilatation	May be a thrill	Loud third heart sound, pansystolic murmur maximum at apex, radiates to axilla, accentuated by turning on to left side
Aortic stenosis	May be slow rising pulse	Narrow pulse pressure	May be displaced	Thrusting apex (left ventricular hypertrophy)	ESM loudest at right sternal edge, ?ejection click, radiates to neck, accentuated by leaning forwards, delayed A2 sound
Aortic regurgitation	Collapsing pulse	Wide pulse pressure	May be displaced	May be thrusting apex beat	High-pitched blowing, early diastolic murmur maximal at left sternal edge, radiates to neck (?+ESM), accentuated by leaning forwards
Pulmonary stenosis	JVP – prominent 'a' wave	Normal	Normal	Right ventricular thrust	ESM maximal at left sternal edge, ?click
Tricuspid stenosis	JVP – slow 'y' descent	Normal	Normal	Normal	Murmur similar to mitral stenosis but maximal at lower left sternal edge
Tricuspid regurgitation	JVP – giant 'v' waves	Normal	Normal	May be a thrill	Pansystolic murmur maximal at lower left sternal edge

ESM = ejection systolic murmur

Example of the presentation of examination findings

On examination, there is no malar flush. There is no cyanosis, or any sign of hypercholesterolaemia. The pulse is 80 per minute, in sinus rhythm and of normal character. The blood pressure is 120/70, sitting. JVP is 1 cm above the sternal edge, and there is no peripheral oedema. On palpation, the apex beat is at the 7th intercostal space, 5 cm lateral to the mid-clavicular line. There is no abnormal impulse, but there is a thrill palpable at the apex. On auscultation, the heart sounds are normal. There is a grade 4/6 pansystolic murmur maximally audible at the apex and radiating to the axilla. It is accentuated by turning the patient on the left side. The features are consistent with mitral regurgitation.

Diabetes

This is an extremely common in both long and short cases, both because it is so prevalent and produces so many physical signs, and because, practically, it is important to know about this condition.

Important physical signs to look for in a patient with diabetes are given in Box 2.14.

Box 2.14. Important signs in diabetes

Skin
- injection site – ?subcutaneous atrophy
- necrobiosis lipoidica
- skin infection

Eyes
- cataract
- vitreous haemorrhage
- dot and blot haemorrhages
- hard exudates (yellow, waxy appearance)
- soft exudates (cotton wool spots – signs of ischaemia)
- new vessels at disc and macula
- retinal detachment

Cardiovascular system
- raised BP
- large postural drop in BP (in autonomic neuropathy)
- ischaemic legs (check peripheral pulses of feet)
- signs of ischaemic heart disease

> **Box 2.14 (continued)**
>
> *Kidneys*
> - uraemia
> - dialysis sites/arterio-venous shunts
>
> *Neurology*
> - sensory distal peripheral neuropathy, glove-and-stocking sensory loss
> - progression to ulcers, Charcot's joints
> - motor neuropathy

Respiratory system

HISTORY

History of presenting complaints

> **Box 2.15. Cardinal symptoms of respiratory disease** !
>
> - shortness of breath on exertion (exercise intolerance)
> - cough (with or without sputum)
> - blood in sputum (haemoptysis)
> - chest pain
> - wheeze
> - stridor, hoarseness

Shortness of breath on exertion

> **Box 2.16. Common causes of shortness of breath and their features**
>
> *Respiratory*
> - pulmonary embolus – acute onset, severe, associated with chest pain worse on respiration, cyanosis, tachycardia, haemoptysis
> - pneumonia – onset of hours to days, may be associated with chest pain worse on respiration, pyrexia, productive cough
> - chronic obstructive airway disease (COAD) – gradual reduction of exercise tolerance, smokers, associated with morning cough, wheeze
> - bronchial carcinoma – gradual onset, may be associated with haemoptysis, pleural effusion, clubbing, hypertrophic pulmonary osteoarthropathy, metastases
> - asthma – acute onset, difficulty with expiration, associated with cough and wheeze, may be worse at night
> - fibrotic lung disease

Box 2.16 (continued)

Cardiac
- pulmonary oedema – acute onset, may be associated with myocardial infarction, orthopnoea, frothy sputum

Other pathological causes
- anaemia

Psychological
- hyperventilation – associated with dizziness, tingling of the fingers, chronic tiredness, anxiety or panic attacks

---

Cough and sputum

Box 2.17. Causes of cough and their features

Upper respiratory tract
- postnasal drip – associated with sinus infection, persistent non-productive cough
- larynx – barking cough associated with hoarseness and stridor; must be investigated for malignancy if persists for more than about 2 weeks
- trachea – in tracheitis, painful non-productive cough

Lower respiratory tract
- pneumonia – productive cough associated with purulent sputum
- chronic obstructive airway disease (COAD) – dry or mucoid (clear, white) sputum, especially in the mornings
- bronchial carcinoma – persistent cough, may be haemoptysis
- bronchiectasis – productive cough, especially with postural change
- pulmonary oedema – frothy white sputum (may be slightly blood stained)
- fibrosing alveolitis – persistent dry cough

Haemoptysis

Box 2.18. Common causes of haemoptysis

- bronchial carcinoma
- pulmonary embolism with infarction
- tuberculosis
- bronchiectasis
- mitral stenosis

Chest pain

Box 2.19. Characteristics of chest pain of respiratory cause

- *site* – central (e.g. pulmonary embolus) or lateral (e.g. rib fractures)
- *character* – usually sharp, stabbing in character
- *aggravating factors* – coughing, respiration, movement
- *relieving factors* – suppression of cough, shallow breathing, rest

---

Wheeze

Box 2.20. Characteristics of a wheeze

- high-pitched musical sound
- on expiration
- prolonged expiratory phase
- causes – asthma, COAD

Stridor

Box 2.21. Stridor

- crowing sound
- on inspiration
- prolonged inspiratory phase
- associated with barking cough and hoarseness
- caused by obstruction of upper respiratory tract
- causes – acute epiglottis, foreign body, laryngeal tumour, croup (in children)

Past medical history

- previous history of asthma or wheezy bronchitis (may point to asthma)
- previous history of tuberculosis
- natural measles or pertussis – may give rise to subsequent bronchiectasis
- previous chest X-ray – useful for comparison

Drug history

- pulmonary eosinophilia (rarely) caused by aspirin or nitrofurantoin

Family history

- asthma, eczema, hayfever or cystic fibrosis
- recent infections (especially tuberculosis)
- smoking history (N.B. passive smoking)

Social history

- smoking – extremely important in bronchial carcinoma and COAD
- occupation – pneumoconiosis and malignancies: asbestos, coal dust, silica; moulds and chemicals may cause asthma or allergic alveolitis

PHYSICAL EXAMINATION

General

- cyanosis and clubbing (Box 2.22)
- nicotine staining of fingers
- tremor (for CO_2 retention)
- lymph nodes
- eyes:
  - Horner's syndrome in carcinoma of the lung
  - iritis in sarcoidosis
- skin:
  - erythema nodosum in sarcoidosis
  - acanthosis nigricans in carcinoma of the lung

Box 2.22. Causes of clubbing

Respiratory
- bronchial carcinoma
- lung abscess
- fibrosing alveolitis
- bronchiectasis

Cardiovascular
- bacterial endocarditis
- cyanotic – congenital heart disease

Gastrointestinal tract
- cirrhosis
- inflammatory bowel disease
- coeliac disease

Others
- congenital (familial)

Cardiovascular system

- tachycardia in infection and acute asthma;
- pulsus paradoxus in severe asthma – an exaggeration of the normal drop in systolic arterial pressure on inspiration. Let the mercury

column drop until the sound is heard only in expiration. Continue to let it fall until it is heard during inspiration and expiration. A range of >10 mmHG may be abnormal.

Chest

Adequate exposure is essential.

Inspection

- chest shape
  - curvature of the spine: kyphosis (forward) or scoliosis (lateral)
  - increase in arteroposterior diameter (barrel chest)
  - prominence (pectus carinatum) or depression (pectus excavatum) of the sternum
- operation scars
- dilated veins on chest wall – superior vena cava obstruction
- respiration:
  - respiratory rate (normally about 15 per minute in adults)
  - depth (e.g. increased in diabetic ketoacidosis or cyclical in Cheyne–Stokes respiration)
  - use of accessory muscles
  - recession: subcostal, intercostal, presence of Harrison's sulcus (where diaphragm is attached)

Palpation

- chest expansion – this may be either measured with a tape (>5 cm is normal), or assessed clinically with two hands on the patient's chest posteriorly with the patient sitting and taking deep respirations
- trachea – assess whether the trachea is central or not
- apex beat (possibly) – may be omitted
- tactile fremitus – should be omitted as gives no added information over vocal resonance

Percussion

- percuss the anterior chest wall (including the clavicle), lateral chest wall and posterior chest wall
- note a loss of cardiac dullness (a sign of hyperinflation)
- compare the two sides
- map out the dullness by going from the resonant to the dull area (see Box 2.23)

Box 2.23. Abnormalities on percussion and their causes

- hyperresonant — phneumothorax
- dull — consolidation, fibrosis, collapse
- stony dull — pleural effusion

Auscultation

- breath sounds — vesicular or bronchial (*see* Box 2.24), normal or diminished
- added sounds — wheeze, crepitation, pleural friction rub
- vocal resonance — patient to say '99' while examiner is auscultating
- whispering pectorilquy — patient to whisper '22' while examiner is auscultating

Performance peak flow

Box 2.24. Bronchial breathing

- indicates area of consolidation or fibrosis

Features
- amphoric quality — like blowing across an empty bottle
- expiratory sound is as long and loud as the inspiratory sound
- gap between the inspiratory and expiratory sounds
- accompanied by increased vocal resonance and whispering pectoriloquy

---

Box 2.25. Causes of reduced or absent breath sounds

- collapsed part of lung
- pneumothorax
- pleural thickening
- emphysema (generalized reduction)
- pleural effusion (absent breath sounds)

Table 2.2. Added sounds, their respiratory phases and causes

Added sounds	Phases and nature	Causes
Wheeze (rhonchi)	Expiratory, musical sounds	Asthma, COAD
Crepitation (crackles)	Inspiratory, non-musical sounds	Pneumonia, pulmonary oedema, fibrosing alveolitis
Pleural rub	End of inspiration and after beginning of expiration	Pleurisy secondary to pneumonia, pulmonary infarction

Presentation of short cases

An example of presentation of physical findings of a 65-year-old man is:

> On examination, he appeared dyspnoeic at rest and centrally cyanosed. He had nicotine-stained fingers, but there was no clubbing. Pulse rate was 100 per minute, and he had warm peripheries. On inspection, there was mild kyphosis and a marked increase in anteroposterior diameter of the chest. Respiratory rate was 40 per minute, and accessory muscles were used. There was moderate subcostal and intercostal recession, with a prominent Harrison's sulcus. Percussion was resonant, with loss of cardiac dullness. On auscultation, there was general diminution of breath sounds, and there is widespread wheeze over the whole lung field, both anteriorly and posteriorly.

You can then discuss the differential diagnoses (mainly COAD and possibly acute asthma).

The abdomen – alimentary and genitourinary systems

In short cases, the instruction 'Examine the abdomen' may involve either the gastrointestinal system, the renal system or, rarely, the genitalia. Even in long cases, it is not always initially clear whether the patient's symptoms are due to diseases in the alimentary or genitourinary tract. Hence, the two systems are included together in this section. Furthermore, it may not be clear initially whether the symptoms and signs are 'medical' or 'surgical' – they may, in fact, be both. Hence this section should be read in conjunction with the relevant sections in Chapter 3.

ALIMENTARY SYSTEM

History of presenting complaints

Box 2.26. Important symptoms of alimentary system

- difficulty in swallowing (dysphagia)
- abdomen pain
- vomiting and nausea
- haematemesis
- indigestion (dyspepsia)
- abdominal distension
- altered bowel habit
- rectal bleeding
- jaundice

Dysphagia

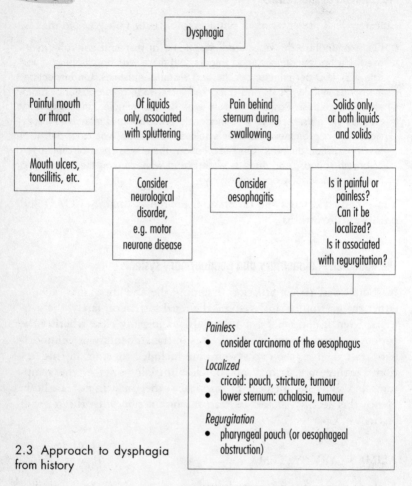

```
                    ┌──────────────┐
                    │  Dysphagia   │
                    └──────────────┘
```

| Painful mouth or throat | Of liquids only, associated with spluttering | Pain behind sternum during swallowing | Solids only, or both liquids and solids |

Mouth ulcers, tonsillitis, etc.

Consider neurological disorder, e.g. motor neurone disease

Consider oesophagitis

Is it painful or painless?
Can it be localized?
Is it associated with regurgitation?

Painless
- consider carcinoma of the oesophagus

Localized
- cricoid: pouch, stricture, tumour
- lower sternum: achalasia, tumour

Regurgitation
- pharyngeal pouch (or oesophageal obstruction)

2.3 Approach to dysphagia from history

Abdominal pain

Box 2.27. Cardinal questions and an example for acute appendicitis

Site initially	Umbilical
Site moved (after, for example, 12 hours)	Right iliac fossa
Radiation	Generalized in late stages
Character	Dull umbilical, sharp in right iliac fossa
Duration	24 hours
Aggravating factors	Movement, cough
Relieving factors	Lying still
Associated features	Vomiting and nausea, constipation

It is important to ask as many of these questions as appropriate, as it will give valuable clues to the cause of the abdominal pain.

Vomiting and nausea

Box 2.28. Key questions

- colour and quantity of vomitus
- smell of vomitus
- frequency
- time of day

Box 2.29. Character of vomit and its cause

Bile stained	Obstruction distal to pylorus
Bitter tasting and yellow	Regurgitation of duodenal contents
Faeculent	Gastrocolic fistula (or large bowel obstruction)

Haemataemesis

Box 2.30. Nature and causes of haematemesis

'Coffee grounds'	Slow upper gastrointestinal bleed
Dark red, with clots	Acute gastrointestinal bleed (varices or peptic ulcer)
Bright red	Oesophageal or pharyngeal source

Dyspepsia

It is important to clarify what the patient means by the the word 'dyspepsia'. It characteristically occurs in peptic ulcers and maybe associated with heartburn and acid regurgitation into mouth.

Abdominal distension

Box 2.31. Possible causes of distension

- fat (obese)
- flatus
- fetus (pregnancy)
- faeces
- fluid (ascites; see Box 2.32)
- mass (e.g. ovarian tumour)

> **Box 2.32. Common causes of ascites**
> - liver cirrhosis
> - malignancy – primary or secondary
> - hypoalbuminaemia – e.g. nephrotic syndrome
> - infective peritonitis

Change in bowel habit

It is important to know what the patient's normal habit is and when the change takes place. Unexplained changes should be taken seriously and investigated (especially considering large bowel carcinoma).

> **Box 2.33. Stool characteristics and causes**
>
> | | |
> |---|---|
> | Black | Upper gastrointestinal bleed or iron medication |
> | Pale, offensive, bulky | Pancreatic insufficiency |
> | Pale | Obstructive jaundice |
> | Blood and mucus | Inflammatory bowel disease |

Rectal bleeding

This should always be investigated.

> **Box 2.34. Characteristics of rectal bleeding**
>
> | | |
> |---|---|
> | Bright red, separate from stool | Anal origin |
> | Mixed with mucus | Inflammatory bowel disease, colonic tumours |

Jaundice

> **Box 2.35. Present symptoms to elicit for jaundice**
> - symptoms of anaemia (in haemolytic jaundice)
> - colour of urine
> - colour of stool (pale stools suggest obstructive jaundice)
> - pruritis is suggestive of obstructive jaundice
> - associated features – severe weight loss suggests pancreatic carcinoma, fever is suggestive of acute cholecystitis

Past medical history

The aspects of the history that need to be determined depend on the presenting symptoms and the possible differential diagnoses.

Box 2.36. Past medical history

- past history of same symptoms or suspected pathology (e.g. peptic ulcer, cholecystitis)
- foreign travel (especially for diarrhoea and jaundice) and immunization
- drugs (e.g. iron causes black stools and many drugs cause constipation)
- past history of blood transfusion (especially for jaundice)

Family history

You may be looking for Gilbert's syndrome in jaundice, peptic ulcer or polyposis coli, for example.

Social history

Box 2.37. Social history

Smoking	Increases incidence of peptic ulcer
Drug abuse	Sharing needles – hepatitis B
Alcohol	Increase in pancreatitis, gallstones and peptic ulcer
Occupation	?Contact with hepatitis, Weil's disease
	Stress (for peptic ulcer)
Lifestyle	?Predisposition to sexually transmitted disease and AIDS

GENITOURINARY SYSTEM

History of presenting complaint(s)

Box 2.38. Urinary symptoms

- frequency
- dysuria
- urgency
- haematuria
- polyuria
- hesitancy (especially in males)
- incontinence (urge, stress or both)
- loin pain
- genital pain

Dysuria, urgency, frequency

Box 2.39. Dysuria, urgency and frequency

Implies disorder of urethra, prostate or bladder
Causes:
- urinary tract infections
- sexually transmitted disease: dysuria only
- prostatic hypertrophy or carcinoma

Haematuria

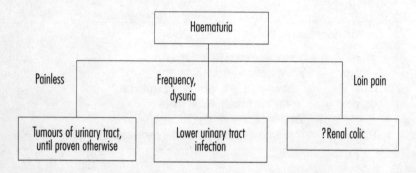

2.4 Approach to haematuria from history

Beware of colour of urine affected by food (beetroot) or haemoglobinuria.

Polyuria
Excessive quantity of fluid. Usually with polydipsia. Causes:

- diabetes mellitus
- diabetes insipidus
- chronic renal failure
- psychogenic

Hesitancy
Usually due to prostatic hypertrophy and, rarely, urethral stricture.

Incontinence

Box 2.40. Assessing incontinence

- duration
- factors – total, urge, stress (cough or laugh)?
- amount of urine lost
- associated urinary symptoms

May be associated with a neurological disorder (e.g. multiple sclerosis)

Pain

- loin pain – may be renal calculus, pyeloureteric junction obstruction (PUJ) or pyelonephritis
- genital pain – may be torsion of testis (acute) or epididymo-orchitis

N.B. Genital pain may be referred to the loin, and vice versa.

Past medical history

Box 2.41. Past medical history – genitourinary system

- diseases with presenting symptoms
- sexually transmitted diseases
- neurological disease (in incontinence)
- past obstetric history (for stress incontinence)
- foreign travel (for schistosomiasis, causing tumour of the bladder)

Family history

For example, of polycystic kidneys.

Social history

- smoking – bladder tumour
- occupation – bladder tumour

EXAMINATION OF THE ABDOMEN

General (Boxes 2.42–2.44)

In the long case, this depends on the presenting complaints. In the short case, if the instruction is 'Examine the abdomen', you can only briefly look for:

- anaemia
- clubbing

- lymphadenopathy (especially supraclavicular, cervical or axillary), as in lymphoma or metastases
- jaundice

and then proceed with the abdominal examination. You can come back to the general features when you have a better idea of the likely differential diagnoses.

Box 2.42. Physical signs of liver disease

- jaundice

Hands
- palmar erythema
- Dupytren's contracture
- clubbing
- flapping tremor

Chest
- spider naevi in superior vena cava drainage area
- gynaecomastia

Abdomen
- enlarged liver
- enlarged spleen (portal hypertension)
- ascites (may be, but is not necessarily, portal hypertension)
- caput medusa (portal hypertension)

Others
- oedema
- testicular atrophy

Box 2.43. Signs to look for in a gastrointestinal bleed

- signs of shock
- anaemia
- telangiectasia of face and mouth (in hereditary haemorrhagic telangiectasia)
- signs of liver disease and portal hypertension
- bruises

Box 2.44. Urinary tract disorder

Ask for blood pressure readings

Abdomen

This should ideally be performed with the patient lying flat or on only one pillow, with hands by the side. Ensure adequate exposure, including the xiphisternum and hernial orifices.

Inspection

Box 2.45. Abdominal inspection

- surgical scars
- asymmetry, suggestion of a mass
- striae
- dilated veins – determine caput medusa (flow away from umbilicus) or inferior vena cava obstruction
- peristalsis
- distension
- obvious hernias

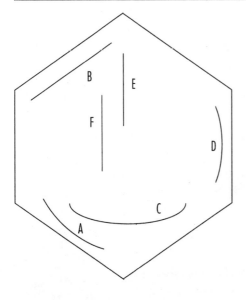

A   Appendicectomy
B   Cholecystectomy
C   Lower segment caesarean section, hysterectomy
D   Renal operation
E   Midline scar
F   Paramedian scar

2.5 Abdominal scars

Palpation

Palpate gently, first asking whether there are any sites of tenderness. Observe the patient's facial expression throughout your palpation.

Box 2.46. What to look for in palpation

- tenderness (Box 2.47)
- masses (Box 2.48)
- liver, spleen, or gall bladder (Box 2.49)
- kidneys (Box 2.50)

Box 2.47. How to describe abdominal tenderness

- severity
- site of maximal tenderness
- extent of tenderness
- guarding
- rebound (omit if guarding is present)

Box 2.48. How to describe an abdominal mass

- site
- size (measure in cm)
- shape
- surface (smooth or irregular)
- consistency (soft or hard)
- edges (smooth or irregular)
- tenderness
- attached to skin?
- attached to underlying tissue?
- ability to indent it (faeces are indentable)
- pulsatile/expansile (e.g. aortic aneurysm)
- associated satellite lesions (e.g. metastases)
- transillumination (e.g. fluid-filled cyst)
- presence of bruit

Box 2.49. Palpation of liver, gall bladder, spleen and kidney

Liver
- start in right iliac fossa and move upwards with each respiration
- fingers should point towards the patient's chest

Gall bladder
- a palpable gall bladder is always abnormal
- in the presence of jaundice, a palpable gall bladder means that the cause is *not* gallstones (think of carcinoma of the pancreas)

Box 2.49 (continued)

Spleen
- start near the umbilicus
- feel for the spleen at each inspiration
- move gradually up and left after each inspiration
- if not palpable, lie patient in the left lateral position, with left hip and knee flexed, and repeat

Kidney
- bimanual palpation
- confirm by balloting

Box 2.50. Difference between spleen and kidney

Spleen	*Kidney*
Cannot get above it	Can get above it
Moves with respiration	Does not move (or moves late)
Dull to percussion	Resonant
Notch present	Notch not present
Not ballottable	Ballottable

Percussion

Box 2.51. Abdominal percussion

- to detect bladder (dull)
- to (roughly) estimate size of liver and spleen
- to ascertain causes of abdominal distension
  - gaseous (tympanic)
  - mass (dull)
  - ascites (1. Dull at flank, resonant centrally. 2. Shifting dullness – locate place of dull percussion, turn patient on side, ascites demonstrated by resonance percussion afterwards at side. 3. Demonstrate fluid thrill.)

Auscultation

Box 2.52. Abdominal auscultation

- bowel sounds
  - increase in frequency and pitch in obstruction
  - absence in paralytic ileus
- succussion splash – to detect obstruction at gastric level; mention but do not perform in exam
- arterial bruit
- venous hum over caput medusa

Check all hernia sites.

External genitalia
Mention examination of the genitalia, although in most exams, you will not need to do it.

Rectal examination
Very important in practice; you must mention it, although you will not need to do it.

Urine examination
Again mention it; it is particularly important if a urinary tract disorder is suspected.

Presentation of physical findings

The above lists formidable, but it can, in fact, be quite short if you stick only to the relevant positives and negatives.

An example of a presentation is:

> On examination, he is deeply jaundiced. There is no anaemia. There is clubbing of the fingers, and two spider naevi in the left side of the chest. There are no other stigmata of liver disease. On inspection, there are dilated veins radiating out and draining away from the umbilicus (caput medusa). The abdomen is not distended, and there are no scars. On palpation, there is a 5 cm of hard, non-tender liver with irregular edges, and a 4 cm, non-tender spleen is palpable. The kidneys and bladder are not palpable. There is no ascites demonstrated by shifting dullness.

Then discuss the differential diagnoses. There are signs of liver disease and portal hypertension.

Neurological system

GENERAL ADVICE

In neurology, it is particularly important that you think about the differential diagnoses throughout and tailor your history taking and physical examination accordingly. Remember that there are many neurological disorders affecting functions that can be elicited from the history, but in which neurological examination can be completely normal (e.g. epilepsy), and there are others that damage structure, which can be localized accurately from neurological examination. You must be selective in your examination. Otherwise, if you merely follow a checklist, you may find yourself spending more than an hour performing the neurological examination alone, at the end of which the patient is tired and frustrated and you are left with a mass of 'results' that may be difficult to interpret.

HISTORY

Try to take history to answer the three questions shown in Fig. 2.6.

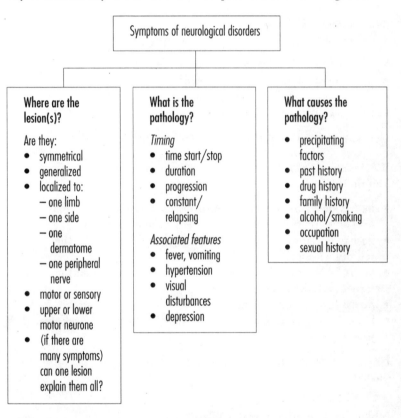

2.6 General approach to neurological disorders

Example

A 60-year-old man is complaining of numbness on both hands. After a full history and examination, you may reach your conclusion by considering the following.

Where is the lesion?
You find that there is loss of sensation, and that:

- it is symmetrical on both sides
- it occurs on both upper and lower limbs, in a glove-and-stocking distribution and is not localized to one peripheral nerve or one dermatome
- motor function is normal

Hence you discover that it a generalized distal sensory loss.

What is the pathology?
You find that:

- it has come on gradually over the past few years
- it is consistent and never disappears
- it progresses slowly but continuously
- there are no associated features

Hence, you decide that it is a peripheral sensory neuropathy.

What causes the pathology?
You find that:

- he has never been exposed to drugs (e.g. isoniazid) or toxins (e.g. lead or mercury) that may cause peripheral neuropathy;
- he has no family history of neurological disorder (e.g. hereditary sensory neuropathy);
- he has a good diet, no symptoms of malabsorption and no reason for vitamin deficiency;
- he has had insulin-dependent diabetes for over 40 years;
- his alcohol intake has been more than 50 units per week over the last 10 years.

Hence you decide that the cause of the pathology is either alcohol or diabetes.

NEUROLOGICAL EXAMINATION

Traditional teaching has been to follow the order of 'higher cortical function, cranial nerves, upper and lower limbs, gait and Romberg's test'. There is no good reason for this other than, superficially, it 'starts from the head and works towards the feet'! You should always adjust the order according to the presenting complaint(s) and perform the most relevant tests first. Moreover, you should have already assessed the gait when the patient walked into the room. You must also be

selective according to the symptoms. However, the traditional order
of examination is: general observations (e.g. involuntary movement
(*see* Table 2.3), higher cortical function (*see* Box 2.53), cranial nerves
(*see* Table 2.6) and upper and lower limbs).

You should notice any involuntary movements that the patient
may have (*see* Table 2.3).

Table 2.3. Types of involuntary movement

Movement	Description	Causes
Tremor	Rhythmical, small-amplitude movements (especially of upper limbs)	Physiological, anxiety (faster) Thyrotoxicosis Cerebellar (intention) Parkinson's (resting, slower)
Chorea	Fast, jerky, unpredictable (especially of trunk and upper limbs)	Huntington's chorea Rheumatic fever
Athetosis	Slow, distal, writhing (especially of hands and feet)	Basal ganglia vascular lesion Kernicterus, Wilson's disease
Orofacial dyskinesia	Tongue protruding, grimacing	Drugs – especially phenothiazines
Ticks	Purposeful, jerky, can be temporarily suppressed	Habit, Tourette's syndrome

Higher cortical function

Box 2.53. Higher cortical function

Orientation
- time – year, month, date, day and time
- person
- place

Memory
- ability to register (repeat after you) and recall a 5-digit number, or a name/address after 30 seconds and 5 minutes

General knowledge (and remote memory)
- dates of World Wars I and II
- name of the current monarch
- name of the current and previous Prime Ministers
- name of the President of the USA

> **Box 2.53 (continued)**
>
> *Attention, concentration (and calculation)*
> - serial 7s (depends on educational level!)
> - simple sums
> - count backwards from 20
> - days of the week backwards
>
> *Language* (dominant hemisphere)
> - expressive dysphasia (comprehension OK, non-fluent) – damage to Broca's area
> - receptive dysphasia (comprehension impaired, fluent with errors and neologisms) – damage to Wernicke's area
> - nominal dysphasia (cannot name objects)
> - dysarthria (pronunciation indistinct, owing to mechanical factors, Parkinson's disease or cerebellar lesions)
>
> *Apraxias and agnosias* (parietal lobe lesions)
> - ability to dress (dressing apraxias)
> - draw a clock face (constructional apraxia; also tests hemianopia)
> - recognize an object (e.g. a key) put in the hand (stereognosia)
> - identify the finger touched without looking (finger agnosia)

Abnormalities of pupils

> **Box 2.54. Pupillary abnormalities**
>
> | | |
> |---|---|
> | No direct light reflex but reacts when light is shone on the fellow eye | Retinal/optic nerve damage, optic neuritis |
> | No direct reaction when light is shone, but the fellow eye reacts | IIIrd nerve or ciliary ganglion damage |
> | Small pupils, associated with mild ptosis, enopthalmos and reduced sweating | Horner's syndrome (e.g. bronchial carcinoma or after surgery) |
> | Slightly large, non-reactive to light, slowly reactive to accommodation, reduced ankle jerk | Holmes–Adie pupil (benign condition) |

Abnormalities of visual field

Table 2.4. Visual field abnormalities

Defect	Lesion	Examples of causes
Total loss of visual field in one eye	Retina, optic nerve	Central retinal artery occlusion
Bitemporal heminopia	Optic chiasm	Pituitary tumour

Table 2.4 (continued)

Defect	Lesion	Examples of causes
Homonymous heminopia (no macular sparing)	Optic tract	Vascular (opposite side)
Quadrantic heminopia	Optic radiation	Vascular, multiple sclerosis, tumour
Homonymous heminopia (with macular sparing)	Occipital cortex	Vascular

Upper and lower limbs

Box 2.55. Inspection and palpation of limbs

Inspection
- atrophy
- fasciculation

Palpation
- tone
- clonus
- power
- sensation:
  - pinprick and temperature (lateral spinothalamic tracts)
  - vibration, light touch, joint position sense (dorsal column)
  - 2-point discrimination, stereognosia (parietal cortex)
- co-ordination (cerebellar):
  - finger–nose
  - heel–shin
  - rapid alternating tapping
  - heel-to-toe in walking
- reflex (use reinforcement if not detected):
  - supinator
  - biceps
  - triceps
  - (Hoffman)
  - knee
  - ankle
  - plantar

Box 2.56. Grading for power

0   No muscles contraction seen
1   Muscle contraction seen, no movement
2   Movement but not against gravity
3   Movement against gravity
4   Movement against gravity and resistance
5   Normal power

Box 2.57. Grading of reflex

+++   Hyperactive
++   Normal
+   Sluggish
±   Present only with reinforcement
−   Absent

Table 2.5. Upper versus lower motor neurone lesions

	Upper	Lower
Muscle atrophy	Absent or minimal	Present
Fasciculation	Absent	Present
Tone	Increased	Reduced
Reflex	Increased	Reduced
Plantar	Upgoing	Downgoing

Gait

Box 2.58. Causes and features of abnormal gait

Hemiparesis	Drags affected leg, inverts affected foot, more contact time of unaffected foot with floor
Parkinson's disease	Difficulty in initiation, small steps, does not swing arms
Cerebellar	Broad based, sways from side to side
Footdrop	Foot hits ground noisily

Romberg's sign

Box 2.59. Romberg's sign

Test: Stand with the feet together, first with eyes open and then with eyes closed

Cerebellar lesions	Tends to fall whether eyes open or closed
Dorsal column lesions, vestibular lesions	Falls with eyes closed, but steady when open

---

PRESENTATION OF SHORT CASES

In the short cases, you will certainly not be asked to do the whole neurological examination. Instead you will be asked to do a specific part of it, such as 'Examine the motor system of the lower limbs neurologically', 'Examine the cranial nerves', 'Examine the motor system of the lower limbs' or even 'Assess the co-ordination'. You should do as you are told initially, but go on to look for signs that may be relevant to your positive findings.

An example of a presentation in response to 'Examine the lower limbs neurologically' is:

> On examination, the muscle bulk is normal, and there is no fasciculation. The tone appears normal, and the power is normal in all muscle groups. Temperature, pinprick, light touch, vibration and joint position sense were all normal in all dermatomes. Reflexes were normal, and the plantars were downgoing. The heel–shin test showed impaired co-ordination on the left side.

Then you should suggest other 'relevant tests' – look for nystagmus, carry out finger–nose test, rapid alternating tapping test and Romberg's test and assess the gait. You should suggest that the lesion is in the left cerebellar hemisphere (although you cannot deduce the pathology at this stage). You may then be asked about its possible causes.

For the instruction, 'Examine the upper limbs neurologically', the presentation may be:

> On examination, there is an obvious tremor present mostly at test in the left hand. The muscle bulk is normal, and there is no fasciculation. There is generalized cogwheel rigidity, which is demonstrable especially in the left wrist. The power is normal in all muscle groups, and in all modalities was normal. Co-ordination was normal, as demonstrated by finger–nose test, and the reflexes in the upper limbs were normal. On examination of the face, it appears expressionless with reduced blinking. There is some blepharospasm.

You should then suggest observing the gait and suggest the diagnosis of probable idiopathic Parkinson's disease.

Table 2.6. Assessment of the cranial nerves

Nerves	Test	Causes of impairment
I	Smell different test substances	Blocked nasal passage, head injury
II	Visual acuity, pupillary reflex (both IInd and IIIrd nerves), visual fields, fundi	Abnormal pupillary reactions, visual fields (see Box 2.54 and Table 2.4)
III	Pupillary reaction, eye movements Damage – dilated pupil, ptosis, 'down and out'	Diabetes (does not affect pupil), carotid artery aneurysm, extradural haematoma
IV	Eye movement (superior oblique) Damage – diploplia on downward gaze, compensated head posture	Head injury, congenital, diabetes
V	Sensation – face, lip, anterior scalp, corneal reflex Motor – muscles of mastication	Cerebellopontine tumour (e.g. acoustic neuroma), peripheral nerve damage in fractures of facial bones (e.g. zygoma)
VI	Eye movement (lateral rectus) Damage – failure to abduct	'False localizing sign' of raised intracranial pressure (find cause), cavernous sinus lesions
VII	Movements of facial expression Lacrimal and submandibular glands Taste in anterior two-thirds of tongue	Distinguish between upper motor neurone lesion (preserved eye closure, forehead wrinkles, usually vascular cause) and lower motor neurone lesion (cause – Bell's palsy)
VIII	*Hearing* – voice when other ear occluded. Rinnes test (comparing air and bone conductance); Weber's test (tuning fork at centre of forehead) *Vestibular* – vertigo(symptoms), nystagmus (sign)	Conduction deafness – local rather than neurological causes Nerve deafness – noise-induced, acoustic neuroma, temporal bone fracture
IX–XI	Palate and uvula movement: when say 'ah', quality of speech, Cough (recurrent laryngeal nerve) (Also posterior one-third of tongue gag reflex – do not test in exams!)	Recurrent laryngeal – bronchial carcinoma Bilateral – cerebrovascular accident, bulbar and pseudobulbar palsies
XI (spinal accessory)	Trapezius – shrug shoulders Sternomastoid – rotate head against resistance	Surgical damage in posterior triangle of neck, together with other cranial damage in bulbar palsy
XII	Protrude tongue – note symmetry, wasting, fasciculation	Wasting and fasciculation = lower motor neurone lesions: skull-base tumour Upper motor neurone – cerebrovascular accident, multiple sclerosis Damage to XIIth nerve uncommon

Diseases of joints

This section attempts briefly to outline the approach and procedure in examining a joint.

HISTORY

Box 2.60. History – diseases of joints

Main pointers to diagnosis
- duration of symptoms (acute or chronic?, *see* Fig. 2.7)
- how many joints?
- symmetrical or not?
- large or small joints?

Other pointers
- stiffness? (time of day)
- associated symptoms, e.g. bowel habit (for inflammatory bowel/disease), eye symptoms (for rheumatoid arthritis or HLA B27 association), dysuria (for Reiter's syndrome), fever (for septic arthritis)
- past medical history (of joint or extra-articular symptoms, and foreign travel)
- family history (e.g. HLA B27, psoriasis)
- drug history (e.g. thiazide diuretics – gout)

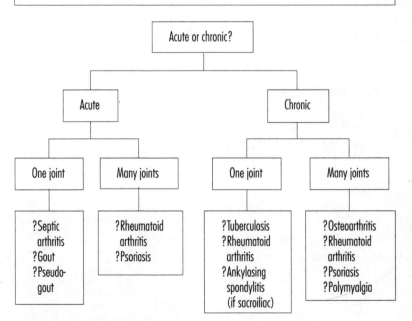

2.7 Approach to joint pain from history

PHYSICAL EXAMINATION

General

2.61. Joint disease – general examination

- eyes – scleritis, episcleritis (rheumatoid arthritis), iritis (HLA B27, rheumatoid arthritis)
- skin – rash (systemic lupus erythematosus), erythema nodosum (sarcoid, inflammatory bowel disease), capillaries in nail beds, psoriatic lesions
- nail – pitting and dystrophy (psoriasis)
- subcutaneous nodules (rheumatoid arthritis)
- hands – Herbeden's node (osteoarthritis), deformities (rheumatoid arthritis)
- ears – tophi (gout)

Joints

Note the pattern of joints involved.

To examine a joint in general, *see* Box 2.62.

Box 2.62. Examination of a joint

Inspection
- cellulitis?
- swelling (suspicion of effusion)

Palpation
- tenderness
- temperature
- swelling – test for effusion if swollen

Movement
- active and passive – detect crepitation and measure range of movement

Others (probably not required in exams)
- stability of ligaments
- special tests in relation to the particular joint

RHEUMATOID ARTHRITIS AND OSTEOARTHRITIS

Table 2.7. Comparison of rheumatoid arthritis and osteoarthritis

	Rheumatoid arthritis	*Osteoarthritis*
Joints involved	Bilateral and symmetrical Especially knee, feet, ankle, shoulder, metacarpophalangeal and wrist joints Usually more joints involved than in osteoarthritis	Bilateral and symmetrical Especially knee, hip and distal interphalangeal joints
Symptoms Joint pain	Worse on waking, improves with activity	Worse in evenings, improves with rest
Morning stiffness	Lasts for many hours	Lasts up to half an hour
Non-articular	Dry eyes, scleritis Carpal tunnel syndrome Pleural effusion Ankle oedema	Nil
Signs Joints	Swelling with effusion Warmth Tenderness Limitation of movement	Swelling, sometimes with effusion Warmth Crepitation Limitation of movement
Hand joints	Distal interphalangeal joints (Heberden's nodes) Proximal interphalangeal joints (Bouchard's nodes)	Spindling of fingers Swelling of metacarpophalangeal joints Ulnar deviation Swan neck or Boutonnière deformities
Extra articular	Nodules, especially on ulnar surface below elbow Vasculitis of nail folds Carpal tunnel syndrome Enlarged lymph nodes Enlarged spleen Anaemia Red eyes – dry eyes, scleritis Pleural effusion Distal neuropathy	Nil

Examples of association of skin lesions with systemic disease

Table 2.8. Skin lesions in systemic disease

Skin lesions	Systemic associations
Malar rash on face	Systemic lupus erythematosus
Erythema nodosum	Sarcoidosis, tuberculosis, inflammatory bowel disease, post-Streptococcal infection
Purpura (generalized)	Leukaemia, idiopathic thrombocytopenic purpura
Telangiectasia on mucous membranes	Hereditary haemorrhagic telangiectasia
Spider naevi (in distribution), palmar erythema	Liver disease
Pyoderma gangrenosum	Ulcerative colitis
Dermatitis herpetiformis	Coeliac disease
Café-au-lait spots, axillary freckling	Neurofibromatosis
Adenoma sebaceum	Tuberous sclerosis
Port wine stain in trigeminal distribution	Sturge–Weber syndrome
Necrobiosis lipoidica, subcutaneous atrophy (from injection sites)	Diabetes

Example of a general medicine long case

HISTORY

Personal details

Name: Alan Jenkins
Age/d.o.b.: 60

Sex: Male
Occupation: Gardener

Presenting complaints

1. Stiffness
2. Difficulty in walking
3. 'Depression'

History of presenting complaints

Well until 2 years ago.

2 years ago – started finding difficulty with getting out of a chair and walking, although he usually managed once he started walking.

Also had difficulty in doing delicate jobs – e.g. used to be good at technology in electronics, found it increasingly difficult and had to give up 2 years ago. Now he finds even tying his shoelaces difficult.

Complained of sometimes feeling stiff, especially in his left leg. He denied weakness.

Met his brother last month, whom he has not seen for a year. Brother thought he was rather depressed, which the patient denied. Sleeps 8 hours per day.

Appetite and weight normal.

Denies symptoms of loss of sensation, pain, headache and vertigo.

Denies tremor.

Past medical history

Appendicetomy as a child.

Had head injury as a teenager while engaged in amateur boxing. Concussed and admitted for 2 days for observation. Gave up amateur boxing altogether afterwards.

5 years ago – had periods of 'anxiety' associated with insomnia. Seen by GP, prescribed stalazine 5 mg tds for 3 weeks.

2 years ago – 'indigestion symptoms' – seen by GP, treated with Gaviscon and cimetidine, which he took for 6 months.

Foreign travel

Nil.

Drug history

Nil.

Allergies

Nil.

Family history

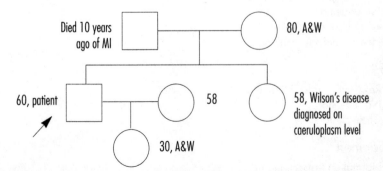

Social history

Smoking, alcohol, illicit drugs
Non-smoker, alcohol 5 units per week, denies illicit drugs.

Occupation
Left school at aged 16 with 5 'O' levels.
Apprenticeship in gardening.
Gardener for the past 40 years.

Social and financial
Lives with wife and daughter in a three-bedroomed house, happy marriage, no financial worries.

Hobbies and interests
Used to go sailing and climbing. Stopped in past 2 years since symptoms started.

Systematic enquiries
Nil of note apart from mild hesitancy, poor urine stream and occasional post-micturition dribbling. No other urinary symptoms.

PHYSICAL EXAMINATION

General

Lack of facial expression. Lack of spontaneous blinking.
No stigmata of liver disease.
No Kayser–Fleischer ring [deposition of copper on cornea].

CVS

Pulse: 70/minute
BP: 120/70
JVP: 1 cm above sternal edge.
No oedema.
Apex beat not displaced.
Heart sounds normal, no murmur.

RS

Respiratory rate: 15/minute
No recession.
Chest clear.

Abdomen

Normal on inspection and palpation.

CNS

Higher function

Normal in orientation, memory, concentration and general knowledge. Writing small and is somewhat illegible.

Cranial nerves

II–XII normal, apart from reduction in blinking. Persistent glabellar tap.

Upper and lower limbs

Mild tremor in left hand, especially at rest.
Tone generally increased, with cogwheel rigidity in the left wrist and lead pipe rigidity in the left leg.
Power normal in all limbs.
Sensation normal in all modalities in all limbs.
Reflexes difficult to elicit but symmetrical. Plantars downgoing.
Co-ordination – finger–nose and heel–shin tests normal.
Gait – difficulty in initiating walking. Take small shuffling steps, with lack of swinging of the left hand.
Romberg's test – normal.

SUMMARY

A 60-year-old married gardener who presented with a 2-year history of progressive difficulty in walking, lack of facial expression and rigidity. There was a history of head injury as a teenager, and there is a family history of Wilson's disease. Examination reveals features of Parkinsonism.

DIFFERENTIAL DIAGNOSIS

[You may wish to discuss the most likely diagnosis being idiopathic Parkinson's disease. Serum copper, caeruloplasmin and a 24-hour urine collection for copper should be performed in view of the family history of Wilson's disease, but this diagnosis is unlikely in view of the fact that there were no symptoms before the age of 58. The history of head injury is again unlikely to be relevant.]

3
General Surgery

General medical and general surgical cases are not always distinct; take, for example, thyrotoxicosis, peptic ulcers and ulcerative colitis. Hence, this chapter should be read in conjunction with the sections in Chapter 2. The sections on the cardiovascular, respiratory and neurological systems are less relevant, as cardiovascular surgery, chest surgery and neurosurgery are generally regarded as postgraduate specialties.

General advice for long cases

In general, you will find that it takes less time to take a history and perform the physical examination than it does in general medicine, as the symptoms are likely to be simple and it is unlikely that you will need to perform a neurological examination.

HISTORY

Personal details

Name: Sex:
Age/d.o.b.:   Occupation:

Presenting complaint(s)

List the complaints briefly, as in general medicine.

History of presenting complaint(s)

For each symptom, ask the questions given in Box 2.1. For abdominal pain, ask where the pain starts, whether it moves and its character.

It is also important to know what the patient would like to be done about the complaint(s). For example, one patient complaining about a pigmented skin lesion may want reassurance that all is well, while another may want its removal for cosmetic reasons.

It is also important to know about the current general health of the patient by asking about the cardinal symptoms of cardiovascular and respiratory disease, to ensure that he or she is fit for anaesthetics should surgery be required.

Past medical and surgical history

The main objectives to consider are given below.

- *Relevant past history* – e.g. a history of past inflammatory bowel disease for a patient with rectal bleeding.
- *Past surgical history* – ask the patient what the diagnosis was, exactly what procedure was carried out and what was found. Also ask about postoperative complications. For example, the patient may have had thyrotoxicosis and a thyroidectomy. However, he or she may also have had the parathyroid gland and unilateral recurrent laryngeal nerve damaged during the operation.
- *Past anaesthetic history* – previous adverse reactions to anaesthetics should be noted, especially the rare but important malignant hyperpyrexia and prolonged paralysis after anaesthetic, so that the anaesthetist is aware of potential problems.

Drug history

As for general medicine, but particular note should be taken of drugs (e.g. monoamine oxidase inhibitors) that may have an adverse effect on anaesthetic agents .

Allergies

Including those to anaesthetic agents.

Family and social history

As for general medicine, and including a family history of *severe* reaction to anaesthetic agents.

PHYSICAL EXAMINATION

Concentrate on the relevant systems. Make sure you have a general impression of the patient's fitness for anaesthetic (a general impression of the cardiovascular and respiratory systems is important). It is most unlikely that you will need to perform a neurological examination.

In cases involving the gastrointestinal tract, you should mention to the examiner that you would like to perform a rectal examination (although you do not need to do so in the exam).

PRESENTATION

As for general medicine, prepare a summary. If the case is postoperative, it can be quite simple. For example:

> Mrs X is a 32-year-old lady who had a subtotal thyroidectomy 2 weeks ago for thyrotoxicosis due to Graves' disease. At present, she is clinically euthyroid on no medication. She has had no postoperative complications.

When you present your case, you have to elaborate on the symptoms leading to the diagnosis of Graves' disease and the present residual signs (e.g. eye signs).

In a preoperative case, the summary may be slightly longer. For example:

> Mr Y is a 60-year-old man who presents with a 1-year history of intermittent claudication, which has progressed to continuous rest pain in both legs for the past 2 months. He has had insulin-dependent diabetes for 45 years, and smokes 60 cigarettes a day. Examination revealed a bilateral carotid bruit, a raised blood pressure of 150/110 and signs of ischaemia in both lower limbs, with absent pulses below the femoral arteries and a right-sided femoral bruit.

Short cases

In general surgery, your short cases are likely to be one of the following:

- a 'lump' anywhere
- the thyroid gland, and assess the thyroid state
- the peripheral vascular system in the leg
- a possible hernia (lump in the groin)
- the abdomen
- varicose veins

although, of course, no list can be exhaustive.

In general, you need less time for each short case as you will be examining something quite specific rather than a whole system. However, you need to be quite thorough. You should refer to the section on the abdomen in Chapter 2. The following sections refer to each of the above likely cases.

SHORT CASE EXAMINATION OF ANY SWELLING

In a short case with a swelling of any site, you should efficiently go through all the characteristics of the swelling and describe them to the examiner (*see* Box 3.1). You will then be asked about the diagnosis. If it is obvious, say the diagnosis straight away, followed by other less-likely diagnoses. If you do not know the diagnosis, you can use both the anatomical and the pathological sieves (*see* Boxes 3.2 and 3.3) to list the differential diagnoses.

Box 3.1. Examination and description of any 'lumps'

- position – where is it?
- size – measure with a ruler if necessary
- shape
- colour
- tenderness
- punctum (e.g. sebaceous cyst)
- attachment to overlying skin?
- attachment to underlying structures?
- consistency – soft or hard?
- fluctuance (test with two fingers; fluid-filled cyst or lipoma)
- margin – regular or irregular?
- transillumination
- associated swelling (e.g. metastases or surrounding lymph nodes)

Box 3.2. Anatomical sieve

- skin (e.g. melanoma, squamous cell carcinoma)
- fat (e.g. lipoma)
- blood vessels (e.g. aneurysm, angioma)
- nerve (e.g. neuroma)
- muscle (e.g. muscle tumour)
- connective tissue (e.g. sarcoma)
- bone (e.g. osteoma)
- gland (parotid gland enlargement, thyroid gland) etc.

Box 3.3. Pathological sieve

- infectious
- inflammatory
- neoplastic
- endocrine
- metabolic
- traumatic
- degenerative
- autoimmune
- physiological (e.g. hypertrophy)

THYROID GLAND

Box 3.4. History – thyroid gland

History of presenting complaint(s)
- weight loss (hyper) or weight gain (hypo)
- diarrhoea (hyper) or constipation (hypo)
- heat intolerance (hyper) or cold intolerance (hypo)
- sweaty (hyper)
- change in voice (hypo)
- tremor (hyper)
- tiredness (hypo)
- neck swelling

Past medical history
- thyroid disease, treatment with drugs, radioactive iodine or surgery

Family history
- Graves' or Hashimoto's disease

Box 3.5. Physical examination of the thyroid gland

Inspection
- size
- shape – is it symmetrical?
- does it move on swallowing? (You *must* ask for a glass of water for the patient during the examination)

Palpation (from behind while the patient is seated)
- confirm size
- confirm mobility with swallowing
- consistency – smooth or nodular?
- thrill (large blood flow)

Auscultation
- bruit

Box 3.6. Examination of associated features of the thyroid gland

Thyroid status
- facial – dry coarse skin (hypo)
- hands – hot and sweaty (hyper)
- tremor – (hyper)
- pulse – bradycardia (hypo), tachycardia or atrial fibrillation (hyper)
- reflex – brisk (hyper), slow relaxing (hypo)

Box 3.6 (continued)

Signs of autoimmune thryroid disease
- eye signs – exophthalmos, lid lag, lid retraction, chemosis (oedema of conjunctiva)
- pretibial myxoedema

PERIPHERAL VASCULAR AND VENOUS SYSTEMS

Box 3.7. History – peripheral vascular system

History of presenting complaint(s)
- continuous rest pain – severity, aggravating and relieving factors
- intermittent claudication
  - duration
  - distribution of pain
  - claudication distance – flat or slope
  - Can he walk after the pain has started? Is he limited by the pain?
  - Is it relieved by rest?
- symptoms of arterial disease elsewhere, e.g. angina, transient attacks of weakness, visual disturbances

Past medical history
- ischaemic heart disease
- transient ischaemic attacks, strokes
- diabetes
- hypertension
- hyperlipidaemia

Social history
- smoking

Box 3.8. Physical examination

Cardiovascular system
- pulse (rate and rhythm)
- blood pressure
- signs of heart failure
- carotid bruit

Respiratory system
(To ensure that walking distance is not limited by breathlessness due to respiratory disease, but by pain in the legs)

Abdomen
- ?aortic aneurysm (pulsating and expansile)

Box 3.9. Physical examination (lower limbs)

Inspection
- hair (loss of hair?)
- nails (fissuring?)
- skin (gangrene/ulceration?)
- colour (pale?)
- colour changes accentuated by elevated legs, and congestion follows when lowered below heart level (Buerger's test)

Palpation
- skin temperature (cold?) – warm knees may mean good collaterals
- pulses – femoral, popliteal, dorsalis pedis and posterior tibial
- effect of exercise (e.g. by moving legs and toes) on pulses – Do they disappear?

Auscultation
- bruit, including aortic and femoral areas

Others
- test for power or sensation if time is available, but can be omitted

---

Presentation

An example of presentation of the physical finding is:

> On examination, the pulse was 80 per minute, in sinus rhythm. The blood pressure was 140/110, and the rest of the cardiovascular system was normal apart from a soft left carotid bruit. Both legs were pale, which was accentuated by elevation. The legs felt cold, the left more than the right, and there was loss of hair on both legs. There was fissuring of the nails, but there were no signs of ulceration or gangrene. Buerger's test was positive on the left leg. Both femoral pulses were normal, as was the right popliteal pulse, which was unchanged by exercise. The rest of the peripheral pulses in the lower limbs were absent. There was no bruit audible in the abdomen or over any major arterial areas in the lower limbs.

You may then be asked to discuss the possible sites of arterial block.

Venous system

Deep vein thrombosis

- *Presenting complaint(s)*
  - calf pain
  - calf swelling and redness
  - (chest pain if accompanied by pulmonary embolism)
- *Predisposing factors*
  - increasing age

- obesity
- period of immobility
- past history of malignancy
- past history or family history of venous thrombosis or coagulation disorder
- recent surgery
- pregnancy
- oestrogen therapy
- *Physical examination*
  - inspection: redness, swelling, engorgment of the calf at corresponding points on both sides;
  - palpation: is it warm compared with the normal calf?; tenderness on palpation of calf; Homans' sign – pain of calf on dorsiflexion of foot (unreliable).

Approach to varicose veins
Examine with the patient standing.

1. Is this due to past thrombosis? Examine for:
- swelling of leg, calf and ankle
- venous ulcers
- eczematous skin changes
2. Is it long or short saphenous vein distribution?
- long saphenous distribution (90% of cases) – usually *above* knee
- short saphenous distribution (about 20% of cases) – *below* knee, in postero-lateral area of calf from the popliteal fossa to the external malleolus
- both long and saphenous systems are involved in about 10% of cases
3. Where are the incompetent valves?
- Trendleberg test – raise the leg and apply a tourniquet at different levels. If the veins remain empty (or fill slowly) after the patient stands up, there is no incompetent communications below the tourniquet level.

LEVELS OF INCOMPETENCE
- sapheno-femoral incompetence – saphenous opening lies 4 cm below and lateral to the pubic tubercle. Incompetence can be controlled by tourniquet around upper thigh below saphenous opening
- mid-thigh perforator incompetence – cannot be controlled by tourniquet around upper thigh, controlled by tourniquet just above knee
- short saphenous-popliteal incompetence – cannot be controlled by tourniquet just above knee, controlled by tourniquet below knee
- distal perforator incompetence – cannot be controlled by tourniquet below knee

A LUMP IN THE GROIN – ?HERNIA

Box 3.10. Questions for suspected hernia

Presenting complaints
- When does the lump occur? On exercise? On standing?
- Is pain or discomfort present?
- Any vomiting? (?obstruction)

Other history
- history of chronic cough
- childbirth
- constipation
- occupation – ?heavy lifting

Box 3.11. Approach to the differential diagnosis of a lump in the groin

- decide whether it is a hernia (*see* below)
- palpate the testis – if it is missing from the scrotum, the lump may be an ectopic testis
- Is it pulsatile and expansile? (femoral aneurysm)
- elevate the legs; if it disappears and there is a bruit when the patient coughs, it may be a saphenous varix
- feel for inguinal lymph nodes – they are usually multiple

Box 3.12. Suspected hernia in the groin

Inspection
- size of lump when lying, standing or coughing;
- direction – indirect inguinal hernia passes downwards and medially, direct inguinal hernia passes directly forwards.

Palpation
- Can you reduce it?
- Is it below and lateral to the pubic tubercle (femoral hernia) or above and medial to it (inguinal hernia)?
- Is there a cough impulse?
- Can you control the lump by pressure on the mid-inguinal point (if it is an inguinal hernia)?

INTESTINAL OBSTRUCTION

This section should be read in conjunction with the section on the abdomen in Chapter 2.

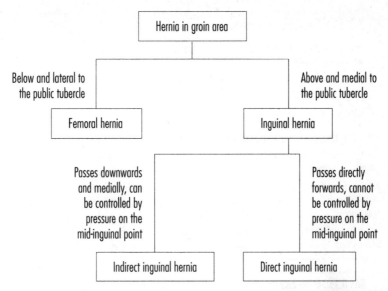

3.1 Hernias in the groin area

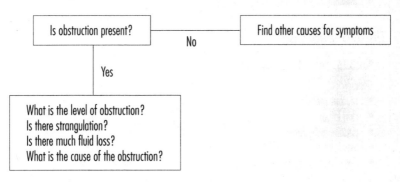

3.2 Approach to suspected intestinal obstruction

Box 3.13. Causes of obstruction

- carcinoma
- adhesions
- hernias — internal and external
- intussusception
- constipation
- inflammatory bowel disease
- hair balls

Box 3.14. Causes of strangulation

- external hernias – inguinal, femoral and incisional
- internal hernias
- ischaemic bowel

History

Table 3.1. History of intestinal obstruction

Cardinal symptoms	High obstruction (e.g. jejunal)	Low obstruction (e.g. colonic)
Vomiting	Early	Late/absent
Colicky pain	In mechanical obstruction	In mechanical obstruction
Abdominal distension	Central, in small bowel	Peripheral in large bowel
Constipation	Late	Early

Box 3.15. Other history

- change in bowel habit (suggests carcinoma of the bowel)
- bleeding PR (suggests carcinoma of the bowel or diverticulitis)
- previous abdominal surgery (?adhesions)

Physical examination

Box 3.16. Signs of intestinal obstruction

General
- mucous membrane – dry?
- skin turgor
- pulse – tachycardia?
- blood pressure – low?
- *dehydration suggests much fluid loss*

Abdomen
- inspection:
  - distension and its distribution
  - previous scars (suggests adhesion)
  - external hernia
  - visible peristalsis – note the distribution and direction
- palpation:
  - rigid or soft?
  - guarding?
  - rebound tenderness?
  - external irreducible hernia?

Box 3.16 (continued)

- auscultation:
  - increased in frequency and pitch: mechanical obstruction
  - absent: paralytic ileus
- rectal examination:
  - important to suggest this to the examiners

Box 3.17. Findings

- rigid abdomen
- guarding
- rebound tenderness
- tense, irreducible hernia

ACUTE ABDOMEN

Intestinal obstruction

See pages 67–8.

Peritonitis – local or generalized

Signs are:

- tenderness aggravated by respiration or movement
- guarding (involuntary muscle rigidity)
- rebound tenderness
- diminished or absent bowel sounds
- shock – tachycardia and hypotension.

Lower abdomen

- *Acute appendicitis – right iliac fossa pain:*
  - initial dull umbilical pain
  - then sharp pain localized to right iliac fossa
  - guarding and rebound tenderness in right iliac fossa
  - associated with vomiting
  - associated with furred tongue and foetor
  - associated with pyrexia
- *Mesenteric adenitis:*
  - especially in children and teenagers
  - tenderness not as well localized as in appendicitis
  - recent cold or sore throat

- *Sigmoid diverticulitis – left iliac fossa pain:*
  - left iliac fossa pain and tenderness
  - associated with pyrexia
- *Salpingitis:*
  - may be unilateral or bilateral
  - usually associated with vaginal discharge
  - cervical excitation on vaginal examination
- *Ruptured ectopic pregnancy:*
  - may be left or right side, pain referred to shoulder
  - history of missed period and recent vaginal bleeding
  - tachycardia and hypotension
  - positive beta-HCG (or pregnancy test)
- *Renal colic:*
  - severe colicky loin pain
  - radiates to groin, testis or labium
  - patient seeks relief by movement
- *Pylonephritis:*
  - severe loin pain
  - associated with rigors and pyrexia
  - associated with dysuria

Upper abdomen

- *Gallstones – biliary colic:*
  - severe continuous right hypochondrial or epigastric pain
  - may radiate to back or shoulder
  - tenderness at right costal margin, detectable especially on deep inspiration (Murphy's sign)
  - may be associated with obstructive jaundice (pale stools and dark urine)
- *Perforated peptic ulcer:*
  - sudden onset of severe upper abdominal pain
  - pain made worse by movement and respiration; therefore shallow breathing
  - tender board-like rigidity
  - associated with NSAIDs
- *Acute pancreatitis:*
  - severe abdominal pain
  - usually (but not necessarily) localized to upper abdomen
  - radiation to back and between scapulae
  - usually associated with vomiting
  - physical examination:
    tenderness, guarding, rigidity of abdomen
    signs of shock

rarely umbilical (Cullen's sign) or flanks (Grey–Turner's sign) ecchymoses

Non-specific site

- *Bowel infarction:*
  - poorly localized severe abdominal pain
  - abdominal distension
  - secondary peritonitis and ileus
  - dark blood rectally
  - shock: tachycardia and hypotension
- *Medical causes:*
  - e.g. diabetic ketoacidosis, lower lobe pneumonia

EXAMINATION OF THE MALE GENITALIA

Penis

- hypospadias – external meatus sited on the ventral surface of the penis
- epispadias – external meatus sited on the dorsal surface of the penis
- phimosis – foreskin thickened and opening of foreskin narrowed

Scrotum

Ideally, carry out the examination with the patient standing while you sit on a chair.

Inspection

- scrotal skin
- presence of both testes in the scrotum
- size of scrotum

Palpation

Palpate the testes, epididymis and vas.

Scrotal swelling

- Does it orginate from the scrotum, and not from an inguinal hernia?
  - Can you feel the root of scrotum between index finger (posteriorly) and thumb (anteriorly)? If not: inguinal hernia.
  - Test for the cough impulse. Positive: inguinal hernia.
  - Test whether the swelling disappears on lying down.
- Is it unilateral or bilateral?

- Compare the size of both testes. If the swelling originates from the scrotum, determine whether it is above, in or surrounding the testis:
  - above: spermatocele (transilluminate); epididymitis (tenderness)
  - in: ?testicular tumour
  - around: ?hydrocele (fluctuant)
  - a 'bag of worms': varicocele

Transillumination
For both spermatocele and hydrocele.

BREAST

History

Presenting complaint(s)
- lumps – site, duration, how discovered, mentrual pattern
- skin changes
- pain
- nipple inversion
- nipple discharge – duration, quantity and colour of discharge, blood
- history of trauma

Past medical and drug history
- history of breast problems
- history of hormonal treatment/contraception

Family history
Breast and gynaecological cancers.

Physical examination
- need to balance the need for adequate exposure against avoiding embarrassment to the patient
- generally need to undress the patient to the waist

Inspection
Inspection is carried out with the patient in the following positions:

- with the hands resting on the thighs
- with the hands pressing on the hips (pectoral muscle contracted)
- with the arms raised
- leaning forward

The breasts are inspected for:

- symmetry
- nipple inversion or discharge
- skin changes:
  - 'peau d'orange' – intramammary lymphatic obstruction by tumour
  - eczematous changes in Paget's disease of the nipple
  - retraction and indrawing of skin: determine whether the mass is mobile over the skin. Immobility may mean tumour infiltration

Palpation
Palpate each quadrant of each breast from the outside edges to the nipple. For any mass detected, note:

- site
- size
- shape
- consistency
- edges
- attachment to the skin or underlying tissue.

Examine the axillary tail of each breast. Examine for axillary and supraclavicular lymph nodes.

Common causes of a breast lump

- *Carcinoma of the breast:*
  - signs: hard lump, fixed in the breast tissue, irregular surface, skin dimpling, dilated veins over the lump
- *Fibrocystic changes:*
  - young women
  - upper outer quadrant
  - changes with menstrual cycle – largest before menstruation
  - rubbery consistency
  - usually bilateral
- *Fibroadenoma:*
  - young women
  - smooth, mobile, discrete lumps ('breast mouse')
  - rubbery consistency
- *Breast cyst:*
  - in young and middle-aged women
  - may be soft and fluctant or hard
  - single cyst or in clusters
  - may be associated with carcinoma so requires aspiration

Example of a general surgery long case

HISTORY

Personal details

Name:	Henry Cutler	Sex:	Male
Age/d.o.b.:	55	Occupation:	Taxi driver

Presenting complaints

1. Left-sided abdominal pain
2. Change in bowel habit
3. Tiredness

History of presenting complaints

A 6-month history of :

- Left-sided abdominal pain, occurs on average once a day, colicky, cannot carry on with his normal activities during the pain; lasts about 45 minutes each time. No aggravating factors but relieved by defaecation.
- His usual bowel habit in the last 12 years has been between once and four times a day. There have been periods of diarrhoea lasting for few months at a time, and he had been suspected of suffering from ulcerative colitis. In the past 6 months, his bowel habit has been alternating between four times a day with diarrhoea, to once every 8 days, with hard faeces. He has noticed blood in the stool twice in the past 2 months, dark red and mixed in with faeces. There is no history of mucous in the stool, no nausea/vomiting, no distension, no recent change in diet and no urinary symptoms.
- Has been feeling tired most days over the past few months. His appetite is steady, but he has had a probably weight loss of 10 lb in the past 2 months.

Past medical and surgical history

1983 – Had periods of diarrhoea. Saw GP and was diagnosed as having irritable bowel syndrome. Given Fybogel Orange. Condition settled after 6 months.

1985 – Diarrhoea recurred, associated with lower abdominal pain. Seen by physicians. Diagnosed as ulcerative colitis after a 'barium X-ray' – cannot recall exactly what was done.

1987–91 – Several episodes of recurrent diarrhoea and lower abdominal pain, associated with mucus in the stool. Was treated with prednisolone and salicylate in 1989; this was stopped in 1990. Last episode in 1991.

No chest pain/heart disease, no diabetes.

Past surgical history

1978 – Nasal sinus washout under general anaesthetic. No complications.

Previous anaesthetic problems: Nil.

Drug history

Paracetamol 2 tablets tds prn for pain.
Colofac 1 tablet tds in the last month.

Allergy

Nil.

Family history

No family history of anaesthetic problems.

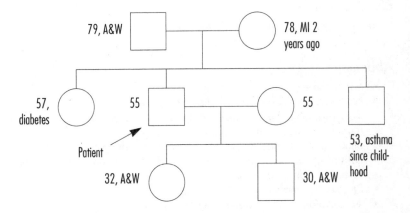

Social history

Smoking/alcohol
Has smoked 15 cigarettes per day in the past 30 years. Alcohol 5 units per week.

Occupation
Taxi driver for the past 30 years.

Social and financial
Lives with wife and son. Wife is a housewife, happy marriage. No financial problems.

Hobbies and interests
Golf.

Systemic enquiries
Nil significant.

PHYSICAL EXAMINATION

General
Clinically anaemic. No clubbing, no lymphadenopathy. Temperature 37.9°C.

CVS
Pulse: 85/minute
BP: 120/85
Rest of CVS normal.

RS
Respiratory rate: 15/minute. No recession.
Chest clear.

Abdomen
- *Inspection* – no surgical scars, not distended, no visible peristalsis.
- *Palpation* – tenderness in left iliac fossa, no guarding or rebound. A 7 cm diameter, hard mass is palpable in the left iliac fossa. It is roughly circular, with irregular edges, slightly tender to touch, not attached to skin and appears to be fixed to underlying tissue. It does not transilluminate, does not pulsate and is not indentable. No liver, spleen or kidneys are palpable.
- *Percussion* – mass dull to percussion.
- *Auscultation* – normal bowel sounds, no bruit.

PR
Not done.

Urine testing
Normal.

SUMMARY

A 55-year-old man with a 12-year history of ulcerative colitis, presenting with a 6-month history of change of bowel habit with alternating diarrhoea and constipation, blood PR and anaemia. Examination reveals a tender, hard mass in the left iliac fossa. There is no sign of intestinal obstruction.

INVESTIGATIONS

Rectal examination.
Proctoscopy, sigmoidoscopy, colonoscopy.
Barium enema.

DIFFERENTIAL DIAGNOSES

[You will need to discuss the need to rule out carcinoma of the colon, given the change in bowel habit and PR bleeding, and that ulcerative colitis can predispose to malignant change. Alternative diagnoses may be inflammatory bowel disease (either ulcerative colitis or Crohn's disease with an inflammatory mass) or, less likely, diverticulitis.]

4
Paediatrics

General advice for long cases

In some clinical schools, there is a separate examination for paediatrics in the finals exam. In others, there is a medical finals, in which you may get both long and short paediatrics or psychiatry cases. In either case, you must be totally familiar with the history taking and physical examination of children, as the approach is quite different from that of general medicine. Students who are just starting their paediatrics attachment may find that they have to change their style of history taking and physical examination from the one used on other attachments.

First, the parents are usually the best source of the history (except for adolescents), and establishing a good rapport with the parents is an essential prerequisite to establishing a good rapport with the child. Good rapport with the child is the only way of being able to examine the child properly. Details such as having a warm hand before performing a physical examination are vital.

Second, one cannot expect to examine children in a 'standard textbook' fashion. For example, you cannot rely on examining the abdomen with the child lying flat on the bed. When examining the cardiovascular system, you cannot always expect to leave auscultation to the last! In fact, you should develop your own technique for maximizing the opportunity to examine the child in the given time; there is no fixed prescription. For example, when the child is sleeping, you should start off listening to the heart, observing the respiratory rate, gently feel the fontanelles (if appropriate) and perhaps feel the abdomen before the child wakes up and cries, when the opportunity of performing these examinations is lost. Therefore you should sometimes be prepared to examine the child before you take the history fully.

Third, establishing a rapport with the child only comes with practice. It is best to have a variety of strategies. If possible, it is best to use techniques that will facilitate the relationship with the child at the same time as performing part of the examination. For example, giving raisins for the child to pick up may establish a rapport as well as test vision and fine motor skills.

Fourth, much of the examination of the child comes from *observation* itself without actually touching the child. The gait of the child allows the diagnosis of hemiplegia to be made more easily than does detailed neurological examination. Listening to the conversation between the child and the mother tells us more about language development than does asking the child direct questions. Watching the child playing with cubes is sometimes more informative than is asking the child to do certain tasks. Hence, at times when the child is protesting and when physical examination appears impossible, do *not* struggle with the child as this will only worsen the situation. Sit back and observe.

Fifth, the history taking and examination must be appropriate to the age of the child. Adolescents may be interviewed before their parents are seen; the techniques for gaining their co-operation are different. The older the child, the more appropriate it is to follow the same routine as in adult medicine. For example, examining a child under the age of 5 years is almost always best done on mother's lap, while examining a child of 13 would be best carried out on the bed, as for an adult.

Sixth, the fact that the history and physical examination need to be flexible means that you must be totally familiar with what is required in the history and examination, so that you know how to complete the history taking and examination without missing anything vital. However, you should write up your notes at the end in the usual order. This will allow you to present the case fluently.

Seventh, if the situation does not allow you to perform a certain part of the physical examination, say so in your presentation. You will not be penalized for this if the examiners find that the child is indeed difficult to examine. However, you will be penalized if you do not mention that you have tried.

Last, it is very important to be familiar with one set of equipment, especially for developmental assessment. Bring your own equipment if possible. For example, if you are familiar with testing fine motor skills by the use of 1 in cubes, and have memorized the relevant developmental milestones, bring the cubes to the examination. There may be other equipment (e.g. cubes larger than 1 in) provided that is equally valid when testing for the relevant developments, but you may not remember the appropriate milestones! Similarly, when you are asked to test for squints in short cases, your examination would be more fluent if you have your own pen torch available while you have the attention of the child. A list of equipment you may consider bringing is given on page 85. You should decide beforehand on your own list.

The following looks lengthy. However, it is not difficult to complete your long case in 1 hour if you know what you are looking for and concentrate on the important points.

HISTORY

Personal details

Name: Sex:
Age (in years and months):

Presenting complaints

This comprises a list of symptoms from the child or the parents, or abnormal behaviour that parents observe, and the i.v. duration.

History of presenting complaint(s)

Details of symptoms (as in Box 2.1), and important relevant negative symptoms.

How the child is feeding at the present is important in all young children.

Birth history

The younger the child, the more important this is.

- place of birth
- gestation
- mode of delivery (vaginal, forceps, caesarean section)
- problems during delivery
- any resuscitation required
- any need for treatment in SCBU, oxygen or ventilation
- birthweight
- any history of neonatal fits
- breast or bottle feeding

Immunization history

BCG at birth
Diphtheria, pertussis, tetanus and polio (write, for example, DPT, polio ×3)
Haemophilus type B immunization (Hib)
Measles, mumps and rubella (write, for example, 'MMR √')

Past medical history

Any past illnesses, with dates and treatment.

Drugs and allergies

Developmental history

This depends on the presenting complaints and past medical history. For example, if there is history of immaturity, neonatal fits, meningitis, etc., developmental history should be recorded in detail. If there is no relevant history and parents are satisfied with the child's development, you can just record one or two milestones under each heading.

Record milestones under 'gross motor', 'fine motor', 'social', 'language', 'vision' and 'hearing'.

Family history

Record any hereditary disease and also any disease with symptoms similar to the those with which the child is presenting. (Both parents and child may suspect, probably wrongly, that the child has the same disease.)

Social history

- Who is living at home with the child?
- Who looks after the child?
- Are there any smokers in the family? How much do they smoke?
- Favourite hobbies or interests.
- Schooling – are there academic and/or behavioural problems? Is statementing under the Education Act required?
- (For adolescents) Use of tobacco, alcohol and drugs.

PHYSICAL EXAMINATION

Concentrate particularly on the systems relevant to the symptoms presented.

Growth charts

In some finals exams, the weight, height (or length in children less than 2 years old) and head circumference are measured and given to on a card.

Plot the values on the appropriate growth chart (for the correct sex and age group) and decide the percentiles for each of height, weight and head circumference. For infants, you should allow for prematurity (e.g. for a child born 12 weeks premature, i.e. at 28 weeks' gestation, deduct 12 weeks from the chronological age).

Also plot the birthweight and the weight at any other time that the parents can remember. Remember that the trend of growth is more important than are the current absolute values.

Ask for the parents' heights. Adjust for gender differences by adding 12.5 cm to the mother's height for boys or subtracting 12.5 cm from the father's height for girls. Then average the parents' height to obtain the mid-parental height. Find the centile from the growth chart (at 18 years). This is the mid-parental centile, and represents the child's growth potential.

General

- Is he or she happy or miserable?
- Is he or she well cared for?
- Is there evidence of anaemia, cyanosis or clubbing?
- Look at the fontanelles (if less than 18 months old) for size and tension.
- Check the state of hydration from the mucous membranes.
- Assess pubertal development if relevant to age and complaints.

Cardiovascular system

See pages 85–8 short cases, below, for details for a 'heart case'.

In non-cardiac cases, recording the rate and volume of the brachial and femoral pulses, palpating the liver (for enlargement as a sign of cardiac failure) and auscultating the heart for murmurs is sufficient.

Respiratory system

See respiratory system short cases, below, for details for a 'respiratory case'.

In other cases, recording abnormalities of chest shape, the rate of respiration and the presence or absence of recission, and auscultation of the chest, is sufficient.

Abdomen

Either examine the child on the bed with a maximum of one pillow (for older children) or on the mother's lap (for young children).

See short cases, below, if a detailed abdominal examination is necessary.

Otherwise, it is sufficient to inspect for distension and scars, and palpate for tenderness or masses, the liver, spleen and kidneys, and hernias.

Central nervous system

See central nervous system short cases, below, for details for a 'neurology case'.

Observation of the child is paramount. Formal examination of tone, power, sensation and reflexes is much less important. There is some element of overlap between this section and that of developmental assessment.

In infants, assess the presence of primitive reflexes and whether they are appropriate for age. In older children, assess the gait of the child, both walking and running.

Observe how the child manipulates objects, and look for squints.

Developmental assessment

You will need to incorporate some of the information from the history into your assessment. Assessment is under the five headings of:

- gross motor
- fine motor
- language
- social
- sensory – hearing and vision

You must know some common milestones of developmental spread between the different ages for all five headings (*see* Table 4.1, page 100).

You must tailor your assessment according to the child. Your objectives are to determine the developmental age of the child under each of the headings. For example, if a child is clearly walking with the hand held (i.e. a gross motor development of 1 year of age), it is pointless observing for sitting unsupported (gross motor development of 9 months). You should look for a higher level (e.g. walking alone or picking up an object from floor) until you arrive at a skill that the child has not attained, and then you can narrow down the developmental chronological age under that heading.

Urine

If urine is provided, you should always test it. For example, proteinuria may indicate nephrotic syndrome or urinary tract infection. Glucose in the urine may indicate diabetes or taking steroids, and blood in urine may suggest glomeronephritis.

PRESENTATION

It is important to leave the last 5 minutes for organizing your notes and preparing your presentation. Always prepare a short summary of the case: it may provide structure to your presentation, and the examiners may want you to present it first. In any case, you need to present it in the end.

The summary summarizes the main positive points of the case. An example is:

Mark is a 4-year-old boy who was born with Down's syndrome complicated by a ventricular septal defect. He was admitted 5 days ago with a history of being off his food, vomiting and having difficulty in breathing. Examination revealed signs of chest infection in the right lower zone, and signs of a small VSD uncomplicated by heart failure. He has a general developmental age of 3 years.

You should mention any adverse factors that may have affected your assessment (e.g. the child is feeding, the child is not in a good mood, etc.). However, the examiners may check it for themselves after your presentation, so your 'excuse' needs to be genuine.

If you are presenting the full history first, it is important to concentrate on the important positive points and relevant negatives. Avoid a list of memorized negatives such as 'He had no past medical history of TB, asthma heart disease or diabetes' or 'There is no anaemia, cyanosis, clubbing, lymphadenopathy or jaundice'. You should be able to present the full history in less than 10 minutes. The examiners may stop you in the middle and ask you to concentrate on specific points. Do as you are told.

After your presentation, the examiners may take you back to the patient to demonstrate some aspects of the history or physical examination. You should be thorough in taking the specific points in the history or examining a particular system of the physical examination, even though you have just done it. You should also show professionalism by being courteous and considerate to the child and parents alike. Remember to wash your hands before examining the patient and to wash them again afterwards (to prevent transmission of infection).

List of equipment

The following are suggestions of what you may wish to bring to the exam. However, you should always decide on your own list and become thoroughly familiar with the equipment beforehand. It is true that there will be equipment available in the exam, but it may not be what you are used to; in developmental assessment, items may not be the ones associated with the milestones you have remembered!

You should be able to fit the following in the pockets of your suit (for men) or your bag (for women). It is important to arrange them so that you can get what you want out easily.

For cardiovascular or respiratory system

Paediatric stethoscope.

For testing squint

- pen torch
- eye cover, with fixation target

For growth and developmental assessment

- a flexible tape measure that can also be used as dangling object. (It can be used for both measurement of head circumference and testing infants following objects with their gaze)
- different-sized raisins (to test for vision and pincer grasp) or 'hundreds and thousands' if you can obtain them
- three different 1 in cubes (of different colours both to test naming of colours and to hold the child's interest)
- a paper and a pen (or pencil)

Neurology

You need not worry if you have not got this neurological equipment. It is unlikely that it will be needed for your short cases.

- paediatric tendon hammer
- ophthalmoscope

Cardiovascular system

HISTORY

In paediatrics, a cardiology case is almost always a *congenital* heart disease. In a long 'heart case', you should ask for:

- presenting symptoms:
  - cyanosis or spells of cyanosis (as in Fallot's tetralogy with infundibular spasm)
  - symptoms of heart failure:
    poor feeding and vomiting
    breathlessness
- family history – of congenital heart disease, although only a small proportion of patients have such a family history
- history of maternal rubella and use of alcohol or drugs (e.g. lithium) during pregnancy

SHORT CASES

You should listen carefully to what the examiners ask you to do. They may say, 'Examine the cardiovascular system', in which case you should systematically and efficiently go through the points below. If they say, 'Listen to the heart', you should just listen to the heart.

As stated before, you should be familiar with the following order, which you should follow in older or co-operative children. In younger children, you may need to deviate from it to adjust to the situation, although you should use the order to present your findings.

General

Look for signs of central cyanosis – compare the colour of the lip or the tongue of the child with the mother (or the examiner!). In central cyanosis, the lips and tongue look blue. Look for clubbing of the fingers.

The presence of central cyanosis and clubbing suggests cyanotic heart disease (*see* Fig. 4.1). If the child obviously has Down's or Turner's syndrome, say so.

Pulses

Feel the brachial and femoral pulses together. Note the rate of the pulse and its volume. In younger children (e.g. below the age of 3), note whether the femoral pulses are normal in volume or weak. In older children, note any evidence of radio-femoral delay, which suggests a diagnosis coarctation of the aorta.

Chest

Inspection

- Note any scars (central or lateral thoracotomy surgical scars) suggesting congenital heart disease that has been operated on. A lateral thoracotomy scar may be a repair for a patent ductus or coarctation, or a shunt operation for cyanotic heart disease. A central thoracotomy scar may be corrective surgery for congenital heart disease.
- Note any chest deformities.
- An increased respiratory rate or recession of the chest may indicate heart failure.

Palpation

- The apex beat (e.g. state that it is displaced to the left 7th intercostal space in the mid-axillary line).

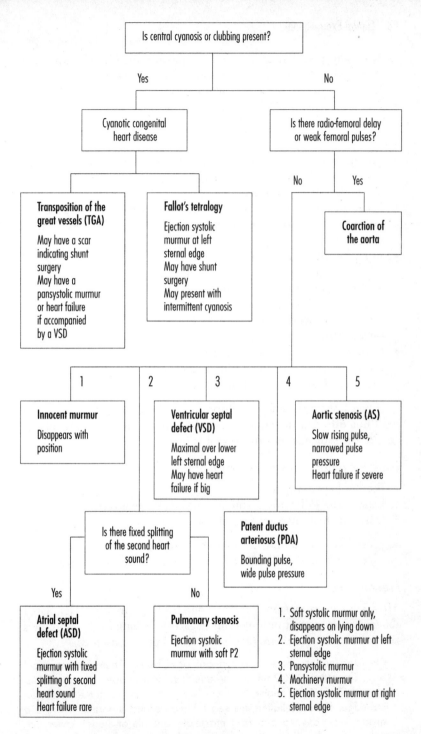

Is central cyanosis or clubbing present?

Yes → Cyanotic congenital heart disease

No → Is there radio-femoral delay or weak femoral pulses?

Cyanotic congenital heart disease:

Transposition of the great vessels (TGA)
May have a scar indicating shunt surgery
May have a pansystolic murmur or heart failure if accompanied by a VSD

Fallot's tetralogy
Ejection systolic murmur at left sternal edge
May have shunt surgery
May present with intermittent cyanosis

Is there radio-femoral delay or weak femoral pulses?

No

Yes → **Coarction of the aorta**

1   2   3   4   5

Innocent murmur
Disappears with position

Ventricular septal defect (VSD)
Maximal over lower left sternal edge
May have heart failure if big

Aortic stenosis (AS)
Slow rising pulse, narrowed pulse pressure
Heart failure if severe

Is there fixed splitting of the second heart sound?

Patent ductus arteriosus (PDA)
Bounding pulse, wide pulse pressure

Yes

Atrial septal defect (ASD)
Ejection systolic murmur with fixed splitting of second heart sound
Heart failure rare

No

Pulmonary stenosis
Ejection systolic murmur with soft P2

1. Soft systolic murmur only, disappears on lying down
2. Ejection systolic murmur at left sternal edge
3. Pansystolic murmur
4. Machinery murmur
5. Ejection systolic murmur at right sternal edge

4.1 How to diagnose congenital heart disease

- Note any parasternal (just left of the sternum) heave indicating increased right ventricular pressure, or a heave at the apex, demonstrating increased left ventricular pressure.
- Feel for thrills. A thrill is a palpable murmur.

Auscultation

- Listen particularly at the apex, left sternal edge, lower left sternal edge and right sternal edge. Also listen to the neck and the back (for radiation of murmurs).
- Listen to the second heart sound for loudness and splitting (soft in pulmonary stenosis, loud in pulmonary hypertension, fixed splitting in ASD).
- Describe any murmur in terms of:
  - its intensity (*see* Chapter 2 for grading);
  - timing: diastolic, pansystolic or ejection systolic;
  - variation with the position of the child;
  - the site at which it is maximally heard;
  - radiation.
- If there is a lateral thoracotomy scar, listen over that side for a shunt murmur (present during both systole and diastole) to confirm that it was a shunt operation.

If you suspect an innocent murmur, ask the child to turn his or her head in a different direction, or ask the child to lie down. Disappearance of the murmur confirms that it is innocent.

Look for other signs of heart failure

1. Feel for hepatomegaly.
2. Look at the JVP (only useful for children in their teens).
3. Listen at the lung bases for pulmonary oedema.

Suggest that you would measure the blood pressure. In most short cases, the examiners will tell you the blood pressure to save time.

Presentation

After your examination, present your findings in the order listed above. You may omit unimportant negatives as long as the examiners saw you looking for them. One example of a presentation is:

On examination, there is no cyanosis or clubbing. There is no surgical scar. The pulse is 100 per minute and regular. The apex beat is not displaced. There is no heave, but there is a thrill palpable at the lower sternal edge. On auscultation, the second heart sound is normal. There is a grade 4/6 pansystolic murmur maximally audible at the left lower sternal edge and radiating throughout the whole precordium and the back.

There is no diastolic murmur. There are no signs of heart failure. I think that the diagnosis is a small-to-moderate ventricular septal defect.

Respiratory system

HISTORY

Presenting complaints

- cough — amount and colour of sputum, presence of blood, intermittent or persistent, diurnal variation (nocturnal cough suggests asthma)
- breathlessness (or poor feeding in infants)
- loss of appetite, nausea or vomiting
- diarrhoea or steatorrhoea (as in cystic fibrosis)
- recent contact with others with respiratory symptoms

Past medical history

- delayed passage of meconium in neonatal period, failure to thrive (suggestive of cystic fibrosis)
- eczema or hayfever (suggests atopic asthma)
- previous bronchiolitis or 'wheezy bronchitis' (suggests asthma)

Immunization history

Especially against pertussis.

Family history

Of asthma, eczema or hayfever.

Social history

Whether there are any smokers at home.

SHORT CASES

You must listen very carefully to the examiner's instruction. The following assumes that the instruction is 'Examine the respiratory system'. If the instruction is 'Listen to the chest', you should go ahead and just listen to the chest! The following list looks long, but in fact 'general' and 'inspection of the chest' generally takes less than 2 minutes.

General

- *Cyanosis* — look at the colour of the lips or tongue of the child compared with those of normal adult. The cyanotic child's lips or tongue looks blue.

- *Clubbing* – this is important in distinguishing between, for example, chronic asthma and cystic fibrosis in the short case. The presence of clubbing generally suggests the presence of bronchiectasis in a child with respiratory symptoms, and hence a diagnosis of probable cystic fibrosis.
- *Fever* – suggest that you would take the temperature.
- *Comfort* – check whether the child appears comfortable and is able to speak in sentences, phrases or single words.
- *Intravenous injection site* – this suggests that the child is receiving intravenous antibiotics.

Examination of the chest

Inspection

Box 4.1. Inspection of the chest

- respiratory rate
- recession (subcostal and intercostal)
- Harrison's sulcus (indrawing of the lower ribs at the attachment of diaphragm)
- use of accessory muscle (especially sternomastoid)
- chest deformities – pectus excavatum or pectus carcinatum (sternum displaced forwards)
- hyperinflation and increased antero-posterior diameter of the chest (indicating chronic obstruction as in asthma), assessed by looking from the side
- timing of inspiration and expiration – increased time for inspiration suggests stridor, increased expiratory phase suggests lower airway obstruction
- stridor or wheeze audible without using a stethoscope

Percussion

- systemically percuss the front, back and both sides for dullness
- look for a loss of cardiac dullness (a sign of hyperexpansion)

Auscultation

- listen for the presence of breath sounds, bronchial breathing, wheezes or stridor, and crepitations
- vocal resonance (listening while the child says '99') is sometimes helpful in revealing patches of consolidation in older children

Perform peak flow

Presentation

In a short case, the most likely conditions are chronic asthma and cystic fibrosis.

Your presentation should be succinct. An example is:

On examination, there is no cyanosis, but there is clubbing of all the fingers. There is a venflon *in situ* in the left forearm. On inspection, the respiratory rate is 20 per minute. There is hyperexpansion of the chest with increase in AP diameter. There is mild subcostal recession, and Harrison's sulcus is seen. The accessory muscles are not being used. Percussion is resonant, with loss of cardiac dullness. There are a few fine crepitations in the bases of both lung fields. I think the diagnosis is cystic fibrosis with chest infection.

CYSTIC FIBROSIS

History of presenting complaint(s)
- failure to thrive
- respiratory – recurrent chest infection or symptoms of bronchiectasis
- gastrointestinal – diarrhoea, steatorrhoea (foul smelling stool, floats on water); meconium ileus (causing intestinal obstruction)
- screened at birth
- diagnosed antenatally or postnatally in those with a family history
- associated with rectal prolapse, nasal polyps, biliary cirrhosis (later) and infertility

Past medical history
- recurrent chest symptoms (wheeze, infection)
- failure to thrive
- delayed passage of meconium or bowel obstruction

Family history
(Autosomal recessive inheritance.)

Examination
- poor growth
- clubbing
- cyanosis (if severe)

Cardiovascular system
(Late stages) Pulmonary hypertension – cor pulmonale.

Respiratory system
- hyperinflation

- is there any use of accessory muscle, or recession?
- crepitations of the lung field

Abdomen

- surgical scar after previous meconium ileus?
- rectal prolapse?

Investigations

- stool – microscopy for fat globules
- chest X-ray
- immunoreactive trypsin (especially for newborns)
- sweat test
- gene identification

Management

- respiratory – postural drainage, antibiotics for infection (especially Staphylococcus, *Haemophilus influenza* and Pseudomonas), and prophylactic antibiotics; may need to be considered
- gastrointestinal – high protein diet and vitamin and enzyme supplements
- psychological

ASTHMA

History of presenting complaint(s)

- recurrent cough, especially at night (wheeze may be absent)
- wheeze
- shortness of breath (if severe)

Aggravating factors

- house dust mite
- animals – cats, dogs
- food – orange food dye
- exercise
- passive smoking

Past medical history

- recurrent bronchiolitis in infancy
- recurrent 'wheezy bronchitis'
- atopic eczema
- hayfever

Family history

- asthma
- eczema
- hayfever

Social history

- smokers at home
- accommodation conditions – damp and cold?
- animals at home
- exercise
- bedding

Physical examination

- short stature?
- cyanosed (in severe attack)
- *no* clubbing
- eczema?
- not able to talk in sentences (during attack)

Cardiovascular system

- tachycardia in acute attack
- pulsus paradoxus in severe attack

Respiratory system

- hyperinflated chest, increased anteroposterior diameter
- Harrison's sulcus

In an acute attack:

- tachypnoea
- use of accessory muscles
- subcostal and intercostal recession

Abdomen

SHORT CASES

The instruction to 'Examine the abdomen' in a paediatric case may involve a range of conditions – a metabolic disorder or thalassaemia with hepatosplenomegaly, a surgical case with an inguinal hernia, liver disease, coeliac disease or renal problems, for example.

The technique of dealing with this instruction is to follow the procedure outline below, but you must be flexible and prepared to follow a certain line of enquiry should some positive findings emerge. For example, finding hepatosplenomegaly would quickly lead the candidate to look for other features, such as jaundice, signs of liver disease, and lymphadenopathy, that might give a cause for the hepatosplenomegaly.

Hence, in contrast to other systems, it is more sensible to examine the abdomen first before deciding what general features to look for.

EXAMINING THE ABDOMEN

Examine older children on the bed with at most one pillow. Younger or less co-operative children can be examined on their mother's lap, and you may not be able to examine as comprehensively as described below. You must have warm hands before proceeding.

Inspection

- Look for previous scars, distension and peristalsis.

Palpation

- You must ask the child whether there is any pain before you proceed. If there is, start with the region furthest away from the site of pain and palpate gently.
- You should be at the same level of the child and watching the child's face while palpating.
- You should strike a balance between exposing the abdomen sufficiently (to include the xiphisternum and at least the inguinal regions), to avoid missing physical signs (such as inguinal hernia), and respecting the child's modesty.
- Perform light palpation in all four quadrants, noting any tenderness. Then perform deep palpation for masses.
- Palpate for the liver, starting from below the umbilical region and gradually moving upwards with each inspiration. You should aim to feel for the edge of the liver on inspiration. The liver edge is often just palpable in children.
- Palpate the spleen with the right hand, starting in the right iliac fossa and gradually moving towards the left hypochondrium. If the spleen is not palpable, you can turn the (older) child to right lateral position with the left hip and knee flexed, and palpate for the spleen again, with the left hand supporting the rib cage. Note the size and edge of the spleen if it is palpable.

- Distinguish the spleen from the left kidney by its position, by the face that you cannot get above the spleen, by its notch, by bimanual palpation of the kidney and by percussion (*see* Box 2.50).
- Remember to check for umbilical, para-umbilical and inguinal hernias.
- You should mention that you would examine the external genitalia, although the examiners will usually tell you that this is not necessary.

Percussion

Percuss to detect an enlarged bladder, to assess the size of the liver and spleen, to elicit a cause for distension and to detect ascites (by shifting dullness).

Auscultation

This is only necessary if obstruction (e.g. pyloric stenosis or bowel obstruction) is suspected.

GENERAL FEATURES

This stage depends entirely on the findings of your examination of the abdomen and the hints given to you by the examiners! The following lists are examples but are not exhaustive.

- hepatosplenomegaly:
  - look for lymph nodes, anaemia and bruises (for leukaemia)
  - note the ethnic origin and facial features (for thalassaemia)
  - look for the stigmata of liver disease (clubbing, spider naevi, liver palm, caput medusae, jaundice, etc.)
  - note dysmorphic features for syndromes with an enlarged liver or spleen (e.g. Hurler's or Hunter's syndrome)
- hepatomegaly only – look for cardiac failure
- enlarged kidney – look for uraemia, ask for the blood pressure and check whether there is an injection site for dialysis (or a shunt in the radial artery)

Neurology

GENERAL ADVICE

The approach to paediatric neurological cases differs from those in adults, although some of the approaches in adult neurology can be applied to adolescents. Remember, one cannot test the joint position or vibration sense of a 3-year-old!

First, the history taken from the parents is extremely important, not only to discover the presenting symptoms, but also to assess the functional level of the child – what the child can do. Second, history and assessment of development are closely linked to neurology – developmental progress is a reflection of maturity (myelination) of the nervous system. Third, the aetiology of a neurological disorder in children is more often due to congenital abnormality, birth trauma or special types of inherited disorder (e.g. Duchenne muscular dystrophy). Hence, the history and examination need to take account of this. Fourth, neurological examination relies heavily on observation rather the tendon hammer!

At a practical level, the cases you will meet in exams are likely to be cerebral palsy (*see* Box 4.4), hydrocephalus (with or without spina bifida), epilepsy (in long cases) and, rarely, Duchenne muscular dystrophy.

HISTORY

The considerations listed in Box 4.2 are particularly important.

Box 4.2. History – neurology

- parental concern at present
- associated features – fits, feeding, behaviour
- birth and postnatal problems (including postnatal jaundice)
- detailed developmental history (especially auditory and visual)
- past medical history (including febrile convulsions and surgical procedures, such as ventriculo-peritoneal (VP) shunt insertion)
- immunization (especially against pertussis and measles)
- family history (e.g. Duchenne muscular dystrophy, tuberous sclerosis)
- social history:
  - who looks after the child at home?
  - professional support – physiotherapist, occupational therapist, social worker
  - educational psychologist, etc.
  - schooling – special or mainstream, remedial help, statements under the Education Act
  - siblings – their reaction

PHYSICAL EXAMINATION

General

- skin lesions (e.g. ashleaf depigmentation (for tuberous sclerosis))
- squints
- surgical scars (e.g. on back for spina bifida myelomeningocele, AP shunt for hydrocephalus (Box 4.3)
- head circumference (particularly important in hydrocephalus in young children)
- fixed talipes (clubfoot) in spina bifida
- contractures (e.g. achilles tendon) in cerebral palsy
- protection helmet (indicating that the child has epilepsy)
- (signs of child abuse)

Box 4.3. VP shunts

Failure to empty and fill	Totally blocked
Empties OK, fills slowly	Partially blocked

Developmental assessment

Full assessment, including functional level (e.g. can the child feed and dress him/herself?).

Neurological assessment

In adolescents, you can use some of the approaches used in general medicine.

Young infants
Stand back and observe:

- general posture – poor head control may mean hypotonia, flexed elbows and plantar flexion may mean hypertonia
- persistent primitive reflex (e.g. asymmetrical tonic neck reflex or grasp reflex – persistence beyond 6 months is abnormal)
- abnormal fisting
  scissoring of the legs (especially when held) may mean spastic diplegia
- which limbs appear to move most?
- note involuntary movements (athetosis or dystonia)

Then you may examine tone, reflexes and fundi, in addition to carrying out a full developmental assessment.

Older children

- General posture – hemiparesis would be associated with fisting of one hand and a relatively fixed, flexed elbow.
- Gait – characteristic hemiplegic gait, with 'winging' of the affected arm. You can also look at the sole of the shoe for the pattern of wear and tear.
- Ask the child to run, walk on tiptoe or walk toe-to-heel. The 'winging' (lifting higher) of the affected arm is more obvious in hemiplegia.
- Test for hand, foot and eye preference.
- (For a child suspected of Duchenne muscular dystrophy – proximal muscle weakness) Ask the child to sit down on the floor and get up. He may need to 'climb with his hands up his legs' (Gower's sign).

Then you can proceed with the relevant examinations of tone, power and reflexes.

Box 4.4. Classification of cerebral palsy

- spastic:
  – hemiparesis (one side of body)
  – quadriparesis (all four limbs)
  – diplegia (both legs)
- athetoid
- ataxic
- mixed

PRESENTATION

An example of presenting the neurological findings (without a developmental assessment) of a 10-year-old boy) may be:

> He was alert and attentive. He wore a protection helmet. He had abnormal fisting of his right hand and appeared to have left hand preference. He had a characteristic right hemiplegic gait, with his right foot inverted and circumducted, and with winging of his right arm. The winging was more pronounced when he attempted to walk heel-to-toe. On examination, he had increased tone on his right side, in his upper more than his lower limb. He had full power in all limbs, and all his reflexes were increased on the right compared with the left. The plantar reflexes were equivocal.

You may comment that you would like to do a visual field examination (to exclude right hemianopia). You will conclude that the boy has right hemiplegia, probably due to cerebral palsy. You may then be asked the causes of the cerebral palsy.

Developmental assessment

GENERAL ADVICE

Different paediatricians adopt different styles and methods of performing developmental assessments. It may appear confusing to a student.

The key lies in developing *your own* style and practising it again and again until you become familiar with your own chosen method.

Students also often get disheartened by the enormous lists of developmental milestones. Many attempt to learn them all, only to get hopelessly confused. The key lies on making up a short list of the milestones that seem natural to you, spread evenly between the four main areas of development and all age groups, and which can be relatively easy to observe in exam situations (e.g. Table 4.1). You should then learn this short list thoroughly, so that you can easily recall the milestones for a specific area at a particular age.

Your performance in a short case will appear smoother and more efficient if you can be flexible and assess all four areas of development at the same time, depending on the circumstances. For example, you may offer a 7-month-old child a raisin from the side while he is sitting unsupported. If he can pick it up with good pincer grasp without losing balance, you can immediately deduce that, 'He can sit unsupported with pivoting, he had a good pincer grasp, and his vision appears grossly normal'. You have thus assessed three areas of development at the same time.

Your objectives should be to narrow down the developmental age of the child in each area of development. For example, if you find that a child can sit unsupported (i.e. about 8 months gross motor development), you are wasting your time testing for head control! You should test for higher levels of development (e.g. standing alone or walking with a hand held) until you can find a milestone that the child has not achieved. Then you can estimate the present developmental age for gross motor skills.

When describing a milestone, you must be very precise. For example, 'He can climb upstairs' is not sufficient. You should specify, 'He can go upstairs one foot per step and down the stairs two feet per step, while holding on to the rail'.

Table 4.1. Developmental assessment (a deliberately restricted list that can be demonstrated in exam situations)

Age	Gross motor	Fine motor	Social	Language
6 weeks	Lifts head 45° in the prone position	Follows dangling object past the midline	Smiles at mother	Vocalizes laughs
4 months	Minimal head lag when pulled to sitting position	Reaches out for objects Follows objects through 180°	Interested	Turns to voice Imitates speech voice
6 months	Sits with support	Palmar grasp of toys, which are put to mouth		
9 months	Sits unsupported	Thumb–finger grasp	Starts stranger anxiety Can play pat-a-cake	Says 'dad' or 'mum' Responds to distraction (see below)
1 year	Walks with a hand held Stands alone momentarily	Index and pincer grasp	Object permanence Waves goodbye	Two words with meaning Understands simple commands
18 months	Walks alone steadily	Tower of three cubes Scribbles	Drinks from a cup	10 recognizable words
2 years	Runs, walks up and down stairs two feet per step	Tower of six cubes Vertical and horizontal lines	Uses a spoon	Two-word phrases Says more than 40 words
3 years	Walks upstairs one foot per step	Imitates a bridge and can copy a circle	Dresses with help	Talks in sentences Can give own name
4 years	Walks downstairs one foot per step	Builds a step with 6 cubes Copies a square	Dresses alone	Recognize three or four colours
5 years	Hops	Copies triangle	Washes and dries face	Fluent speech

HISTORY

In a developmental assessment, the history from the parents is extremely important. Any concerns that the parents have are usually justified. This is especially true for hearing and visual developments. Hence in the long case, one should start with, 'Are there any concerns about his or her developments so far?'

The objectives should be to obtain enough information on all five areas of development – gross motor, fine motor, language, social and sensory (hearing and vision). Of course, normal hearing and visual development is essential for language and fine motor development respectively. If an area of development appears normal, one needs not go into every milestone. On the other hand, if there is suspicion of delay in any particular area, that area should be explored in detail to uncover the stage at which the delay has occurred.

EXAMINATION

In short cases, the examiners may or may not allow you to ask the parents questions. Always mention that you would like to do so.

You should begin by simply observing the child for some time. Much can be deduced about the child's development in the four areas, and you can comment on the milestones to the examiner while you are observing. An example of what you can say of a 1-year-old child in the first minute of your observation is:

> The child is able to walk with a hand held. He has a fine pincer grasp. He is able to say at least four words with meaning, and he shows stranger anxiety.

If the child is apprehensive or appears unco-operative, spending a longer time observing, especially the interaction with the parents, may be the best strategy. Alternatively, you can get the parents to ask the child to do the tasks you have in mind.

The subsequent approaches should start with the least intrusive assessments first. The following are suggestions only.

Less than 6 months old

- Dangle an object (e.g. your flexible tape measure) in front of the child and assess whether the child can follow the object from side to side, vertically and in a circle.
- Assess whether the child reaches out for the object. If so, see whether he or she puts it to the mouth, and assess the grasp (ulnar or palmar).

- Assess any noises the child makes.
- Leave assessments of head control until the end. Assess the grasp reflex, and then pull the child up from supine position and assess the head lag.

6 months to 1 year old

- Offer raisins (or 'hundreds and thousands') and assess the grasp (pincer grasp?) and vision.
- During this period, keep talking to the child and assess any noises or vocalizations that the child can make.
- Note any signs of stranger anxiety.
- Offer the child a 1in cube. Note whether it is put to the mouth or transferred to the other hand. If it is dropped, see whether the child will look for it on the floor (object permanence). Then offer a second 1in cube. Assess whether the child can hold the two cubes together. Note whether he or she will bang the two bricks together.
- Assess during this time how steadily the child is sitting. Note whether the back is straight or curved. Test whether the child can sit unsupported and, if so, how steadily (test whether he or she can pick up an object placed behind). Then assess whether the child can stand with support or alone, or walk.
- Try to wave goodbye to the child – can he or she do the same?

Over 18 months old

Use the following methods (in any order):

- building with cubes
- copying and imitating using a pencil and paper
- testing speech and understanding by talking to him or her and using picture books
- seeing how well the child can walk (with or without a hand held), run and climb stairs (up or down), holding the rail or not, one or two feet per step

PRESENTATION

You should present your findings succinctly under each developmental area and give an estimated developmental age. Then give your conclusion as to whether the child's development is normal, delayed in one area or globally delayed. One example of a presentation is:

She can sit unsupported with good pivoting for 5 minutes and can be held standing. However, she cannot stand alone or walk with a hand held. I think her gross motor development age is about 9–10 months.

In her fine motor development, she bangs two cubes together and has a good pincer grasp. She cannot yet build a tower of two cubes or scribble. I think her fine motor development is about 12 months. She also demonstrates appropriate visual development.

Socially, she showed stranger anxiety, was able to wave goodbye and showed object permanence. She cannot yet use a spoon or help with dressing. I think her social level of development is about 12 months.

She says 'dad', 'mum' and 'car' appropriately. Her speech development is equivalent to at least 12 months old.

As her chronological age is 11 months, I conclude that her development is normal.

An example for delayed development is:

In his gross motor development, he can run without falling and walk up and downstairs two feet per step holding on to a rail, but he cannot walk upstairs one foot per step. I think his gross motor development is of around 2 years old.

He can build a tower of seven cubes and can copy a vertical and horizontal line. He cannot yet imitate a circle. I think that his fine motor development is equivalent to about 2 years.

In his speech, he can only say 'mum' and 'dad' indistinctly, and I could not detect any other words during the interview. I would like to ask the parents about his speech at home, but I suspect that his speech development level is at about 10 months.

Socially, he can drink from a cup using two hands and he can use a spoon. He can take off his coat with help. His social developmental age is around 2 years.

His chronological age is 2 years. I think he has an isolated speech delay. This may be due to poor hearing, and I should like to test his hearing and look for signs of glue ear.

DISTRACTION TEST

The distraction test is a widely used screening test for hearing, usually performed at 8 months of age. As they are mostly carried out by health visitors, doctors have often lost their skills in this test. You will be expected to know the principles of this test and may very occasionally be asked to demonstrate it in short cases.

The test involves observing the child's ability to localize test sounds of both high and low frequency presented 1m from each side. It is important to eliminate the possibility of the child responding to cues (e.g. movement) other than the sound presented, and also the possibility that the child becomes so interested in other objects that he or she does not respond even though the hearing is intact. The procedures are as follows:

1. Three adults are required for this test. Sit the child on mother's knee, ask the examiner to be the distracter and present the sound yourself.
2. Make sure that the room is as quiet as possible. Close the door! Make sure that the child cannot see your shadow when you move behind him or her.
3. Ask the examiner to distract the child using a large attractive object (such as a teddy bear). You should stay quietly behind the child.
4. When the child's attention has been caught for some time, the examiner will gradually take away or cover up the object, so that the child's concentration to other sound is at a maximum. You should then, within a second or two, present your test sound.
5. The test sound should be presented about 1 m to the side at the child's ear level. The particular test sound used varies between centres. Manchester rattles may be used and rubbing tissue paper or a soft 's' may be used for high-frequency sounds. A soft 'oo' may be used as a low-frequency sound. There are new, specialized pieces of equipment that emit sound of a known loudness and frequency.
6. Congratulate the child if he or she responds.
7. A positive response is if the child localizes the source of sound by turning his or her head. The test is usually done three times, and a response of at least two of out of three represents a pass.
8. The test is repeated with both low- and high-frequency sounds on both sides.

Squints

SHORT CASES

Squints are common short cases in finals. Not only are they common, but it is also important to diagnose them early in practice to prevent amblyopia (lazy eye), with irreversible loss of visual acuity later on in life.

Make sure that it is not a paralytic squint (i.e. ensure that each eye has a full range of movement when the other is covered).

TRUE SQUINT OR PSEUDO-SQUINT?

Epicanthic folds, for example, may mimic a convergent squint. More-over, both conditions can be present together. Distinguish between them using corneal reflection test.

Using a pen torch, shine a light from a distance (e.g. at least 1 m away) and notice the reflection in each cornea. For example:

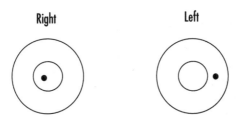

may indicate a left convergent squint or a right divergent squint.

If the reflections are central in both eyes, there is no squint, and the appearance is a pseudo-squint.

COVER TEST

Ask the child to look at your fixation target (e.g. picture or pen torch) held at least 1m away. Cover one eye (e.g. the right eye) while you observe the other (left eye). If there is movement, the covered (right) eye is the usual fixating eye, and the left eye is the squinting eye. If there is no movement, the left eye is the usual fixating eye.

Now uncover the right eye, and observe the uncovered (right) eye. If there is movement, this confirms that the right eye is the fixating eye.

In alternating squints, either eye may be the fixating eye.

ALTERNATIVE COVER TEST

Latent squint may not be revealed by the cover test. Alternate between covering the right and the left eye every 2 seconds, while the child fixes on a picture or pen torch held 1 m away. Latent squints may be revealed by movement of the eye when covered/uncovered.

Common syndromes seen in exams

DOWN'S SYNDROME (TRISOMY 21)

Box 4.5. Physical signs of Down's syndrome

General
- hypotonia
- short stature
- developmental delay

Head and face
- delayed closure of the anterior fontanelle
- may be a third fontanelle
- upward sloping palpebral fissures
- Brushfield spots (white dots like a clock face in the iris)
- epicanthic folds
- may be a squint

Hands and feet
- incurving fifth finger (clinodactyly)
- single palmar crease
- wide gap between first and second toes

Cardiovascular system
- increased incidence of atrioventicular canal defect, patent ductus arteriosus
- VSD and Fallot's tetralogy

Gastrointestinal
- increased rate of duodenal atresia and Hirschsprung's disease

---

TURNER'S SYNDROME (XO)

Box 4.6. Physical signs of Turner's syndrome

- short stature
- webbed short neck
- low hair line
- puffy feet and hands (in the newborn)
- widely spaced nipples
- 15 per cent have coarction of the aorta
- lack of secondary sexual characteristics (in untreated cases)

NEUROFIBROMATOSIS

Autosomal dominant

Box 4.7. Physical signs of neurofibromatosis

- skin nodules (neurofibromas)
- café-au-lait spots
- axillary freckling
- acoustic neuromas (in some types of neurofibromatosis)
- may be scoliosis
- may be increased blood pressure from renal artery stenosis or phaeochromocytoma

---

TUBEROUS SCLEROSIS

Autosomal dominant

Box 4.8. Tuberous sclerosis

History
- may have epilepsy
- may have mental retardation

Examination
- depigmented patches – 'ashleaf' depigmentation
- papules on face – adenoma sebaceum – from teenage
- fibromata under nails

SURGE–WEBER SYNDROME

- associated with epilepsy
- port wine stain on one side of the face (area of the ophthalmic division of the trigeminal nerve)

Example of a paediatric long case

HISTORY

Personal details

Name: Harry Child   Sex: Male
Age: 3 years 3 months

Presenting complaints

1. Fever
2. Vomiting
3. Cough
4. Poor growth

History of presenting complaints

Mother worried about lack of weight gain in the past year; gives weight as 11.8 kg aged 2 years 3 months (25th percentile), 12.1 kg at 2 years 9 months (10th percentile) and 12.3 kg a few days ago (below 10th percentile). Appetite usually normal, and diet generally satisfactory.

4 days ago, became generally miserable. Went off food and started occasional dry cough, usually in day time. Seen by GP, diagnosed as having a viral infection and advised to take fluids.

2 days ago, developed fever of 38.5°C. Cough becomes worse and sounds productive, and Harry has twice vomited up what looks like green sputum. He is taking adequate fluids but refusing food.

No breathlessness or wheezing. Bowels open once a day. Stools generally well formed, except on a few occasions in the past month when the mother noted foul-smelling stools (although she cannot elaborate any further). Denies headache.

Birth history

Place of birth: Ipswich
Gestation: 40 weeks
Antenatal problem: Nil
Mode of delivery: Vaginal
Resuscitation: Nil
Problems postnatally: Passed meconium at 4 days, nil else
Birthweight: 3.1 kg
Feeding: Breast fed for 1 month, then bottle fed

Immunization history

BCG: Nil
DPT and polio: ×3
Hib: Nil
MMR: At 18 months

Past medical history

Aged 6/12 – Diagnosed as having Haemophilus meningitis, treated by intravenous antibiotics, in hospital for 3 weeks. Failed distraction test and had a mild hearing problem. No other complications.

Aged 1–3 years – Had at least eight episodes of productive cough with fever, treated by GP with antibiotics, except for admission for 1 week aged 2 years 3 months, treated with intravenous antibiotics.

Drug history and allergies

Nil before this illness. Now treated with intravenous gentamicin and penicillin.

Developmental history

- Gross motor – walked alone aged 18 months; now walks upstairs one foot per step.
- Fine motor – mother has no concerns.
- Social – dry by day; uses a spoon and fork.
- Language – said 'dad' and 'mum' at 2 years. Vocabulary now about 50 words and he can just form two-word phrase.
- Hearing and vision – mother notices that she has to talk loudly to him. Vision OK.

Family history

No family history of hereditary diseases. No asthma, eczema or hayfever.

Social history

Parent's ages and occupations:

- Father (29) bus driver
- Mother (28) housewife

Both parents smoke 20 cigarettes per day in the house.
Siblings: one older brother (Mark) aged 6. Well. (Mother has had no other pregnancy.)
Schooling: nil.
Hobbies and interests: nil particular.
Accommodation: lives in a two-bedroomed, terraced house with his parents and brother.

PHYSICAL EXAMINATION

Growth

Height: 96cm
Weight: 12.3kg
Head circumference: N/A
(Plot on appropriate charts)
Mid-parental height and percentile: 176cm (50th percentile)

General

Alert, but miserable. Temperature 37.8°C. Venflon *in situ* left forearm.
Throat not infected. Tympanic membranes normal.
No cyanosis or anaemia.
No clubbing.

CVS

Pulse 100/minutes. Femoral pulses strong. No heave. Heart sounds normal. No murmur.

RS

Respiratory rate: 30/minute.
Minimal use of accessory muscles.
Mild intercostal/subcostal recession. No Harrison's sulcus.
Possibly increased anteroposterior diameter of the chest.
Percussion resonant.
Bronchial breathing at left lower zone posteriorly. Mild wheezing audible at both bases.

Abdomen

Soft, non-tender. No liver, spleen or kidney palpable.

Central nervous system

No neck stiffness. Kernig sign negative.
Gait normal.
Rest of examination not done.

Development

- Gross motor – runs, goes upstairs one foot per step, downstairs two feet per step. Can just stand on one foot momentarily.
- Fine motor – builds a tower of nine blocks. Refused to co-operate with pen and paper test.
- Speech – says 'Car goes'. Used a total of 15 words of vocabulary at interview. Cannot give full name.
- Social – drinks from a cup using two hands. Uses a spoon.
- Vision and hearing – vision normal using 'hundreds and thousands'. Refused to co-operate with STYCAR. Refused to co-operate with hearing test.

SUMMARY

3 year 3 month-old boy who has failure to thrive in the last year and has had recurrent episodes of chest infection over the past 2 years. He presented with a 4-day history of productive cough, fever and vomiting. There was a history of delayed passage of meconium at birth, and a his-

tory of foul-smelling stools. He also had a treated Haemophilus meningitis aged 6 months, which left him with a mild hearing deficit and delayed speech development. Examination confirmed signs of chest infection at the left lower zone, and he is currently receiving antibiotic treatment.

COMMENTS

[In the differential diagnoses, you obviously have to mention cystic fibrosis.

You should mention that you should perform the developmental assessment again when the child is well. Performing developmental assessment when a child is still having an acute illness is often unsuccessful and the results unreliable.]

5
Obstetrics

General advice for long cases

In the finals exam, this is usually assessed by only one long case. In some clinical schools, there are separate obstetrics and gynaecology exams, whereas in others, there is a combined exam in which long cases may either be obstetrics or gynaecology.

The usual time allowed for interviewing patients in obstetrics varies between clinical schools, but is usually about 30 minutes – less that that allowed for medicine or surgery. It is important to be comprehensive in the sections of history and examination that are especially relevant (e.g. antenatal history and past obstetric history) but not to spend too much time on other less relevant sections. Thirty minutes is usually quite sufficient to complete a reasonable history and examination.

It is wise to bring your own obstetric calendar and tape measure and to be familiar with the equipment beforehand.

Note that you may have a case of a normal pregnancy. This is neither advantageous nor disadvantageous; you will still have to take the same history (*see* Box 5.1) and demonstrate your physical examination technique. You may afterwards be asked questions on, for example, the induction of labour or antenatal care.

Box 5.1. Approach to obstetrics cases

When you take the history, ask yourself the following three questions:
1. Is this a low- or high-risk pregnancy? (*See* page 125.)
2. What abnormalities (if any) are there in this pregnancy?
3. What special management is needed:
   (a) before labour
   (b) during labour
   (c) after delivery for both mother and baby?

HISTORY

Personal details

Name: Ethnicity:
Age: Occupation:
Marital status:

History of present pregnancy
Is this pregnancy planed or unplanned?

LMP, present gestation and EDD
Note the:

- last menstrual period (LMP) (i.e. the first day of the last period)
- contraception used before pregnancy
- usual duration and frequency of periods before pregnancy

From the above, work out, using the obstetric calendar, the present gestation and estimated date of delivery (EDD). (N.B. If the duration of normal cycles is significantly different from 28 days, add the difference to the EDD if it is more than 28 days, and subtract the difference if it is less than 28 days.

A rough rule for working out the EDD from LMP is to add 7 days and subtract 3 months, correcting for the previous frequency of periods if appropriate. For example, a woman with a 35-day cycle and an LMP of 5 May 1994 would have an EDD of 12 February 1995 (uncorrected) or 19 February 1995 (corrected for the frequency of periods).

- gestation by ultrasound (if known by patient)

Antenatal care

- date of booking and investigations (*see* section on routine antenatal investigations)
- problems noted, investigations undertaken and treatment given
- any problems in this pregnancy, from patient's point of view

Symptoms of pregnancy
Nausea and vomiting, frequency of micturition, tiredness or breast tenderness.

Plan for feeding
Breast or bottle feeding.

Past obstetric history

For each pregnancy, list:

- year
- gestation
- antenatal problems
- intrapartum problems
- mode of delivery
- outcome – abortion (spontaneous or therapeutic), stillbirth, livebirth
- sex of fetus
- postnatal problems and mode of feeding
- if the mother is blood group rhesus negative, whether Anti-D was given after delivery

Past gynaecological history

List year, diagnosis and intervention for each problem.

Past medical history

This can generally be brief. However, diseases such as cardiac or thyroid problems, diabetes or systemic lupus erythematosus must be recorded if present.

Blood group (if known) and rubella immunization status should also be noted.

Drug history

List both current medications and those taken during and just before conception (some drugs may be teratogenic).

Allergies

Family history

Of diabetes, twins and hereditary disorders.

Social history

- accommodation condition and provision for the future child
- Is the partner supportive? Who else provides support?
- smoking and alcohol history (very important)
- illicit drug history during conception or pregnancy
- financial problems

Direct questioning

You may omit this if you run out of time. Enquire particularly about heartburn, constipation, varicose veins and haemorrhoids.

PHYSICAL EXAMINATION

N.B. Never lie the patient flat, because of the risk of the compression of the inferior vena cava.

General

- evidence of anaemia
- height, weight and shoe size

Cardiovascular system

- pulse
- blood pressure – this is vital
- evidence of oedema – ankle, fingers or face
- evidence of a flow murmur

Respiratory system

Examination can be brief unless respiratory disease is in the history or suspected.

Abdomen

This is the most important part of the physical examination; the abdomen *must* be examined in the following order.

Inspection

Look for striae and previous surgical scars. Note whether abdominal size is compatible with dates. A rough estimation is:

- 12 weeks – palpable suprapubically
- 20 weeks – fundus at the umbilicus
- 28 weeks – fundus half-way between the umbilicus and the xiphisternum
- 36 weeks – at the xiphisternum

Measure (in cm) the fundal height – the distance between the fundus and the symphysis pubis. Generally, this should roughly correspond with the gestation in weeks.

Palpation

Note the amount of amniotic fluid. Demonstrate a fluid thrill if you suspect polyhydramnios. (Ask the examiner to put the edge of his or her hand on the centre of the abdomen while you elicit a fluid thrill.)
Determine:

- lie – longitudinal, transverse or oblique
- presentation – (if longitudinal) cephalic or breech

- number of fifths palpable – (if cephalic) if two-fifths or less is palpable, the head is said to be engaged
- which side the fetal back is palpable

Auscultation
Fetal heart: auscultate with the fetal stethoscope over the position of the anterior shoulder or in the midline if the shoulder is not palpable. Try 8 cm above the symphysis pubis in the midline for a cephalic presentation, and at the level of the umbilicus if you are unsure of the position of the anterior shoulder. If you cannot hear the heart in the examination, it is more likely that it is there but that you cannot hear it! Suggest to the examiner using a Sonacaid.

Central nervous system

Test for increased reflexes and look at the optic fundus for papilloedema and haemorrhages if there is hypertension.

Vaginal examination

You would *not* need to carry this out in an exam. However, you may be asked what you would look for in the vaginal examination.

By vaginal examination you can determine the level of the presenting parts in relation to the ischial spine and generally assess the size of the pelvic outlet. You cannot determine the position accurately until the mother is in labour and the cervix is fully dilated.

Test the urine

This is important and is often asked for by examiners, especially when a specimen is provided. Proteinuria may indicate urinary tract infection or pre-eclampsia, and glucose in the urine may indicate gestational diabetes.

PRESENTATION

It is sometimes wise to present a summary of the case to the examiners to begin with, so that they may ask you to concentrate on some specific areas if they wish. In any case, you need a summary at the end. Prepare the summary by writing it down before meeting the examiners.

The summary should consist of:

- name
- age
- marital status

- ethnicity;
- occupation;
- The number of previous pregnancies and number of previous live births/abortions. This is often abbreviated to, for example, gravida 4, para 1. 'Gravida' indicates the number of times the woman has been pregnant (including the present pregnancy), and 'para' refers to the number of potentially viable fetuses she has delivered. Hence gravida 3, para 1 indicates that this is her third pregnancy, she has delivered one potentially viable fetus and had one miscarriage or termination of pregnancy. If your case is complicated (e.g. pairs of twins or a mixture of terminations and miscarriages), you may prefer to state the exact findings rather than use these abbreviations.
- gestation by dates/ultrasound;
- significant past medical history (if any);
- presenting problems (N.B. it may be a normal pregnancy!).

An example of a presentation is:

> I would like to present Mrs X, a 29-year-old catering manager, gravida 3, para 1, with a 20-year history of insulin-dependent diabetes, who is now 36 weeks gestation by ultrasound. She presented with 2 days of symptoms and signs of pre-eclampsia and was admitted for bed rest and blood pressure monitoring.

Then present the full history, unless the examiners indicate that they are particularly interested in some aspects of the history or examination. You must be sensitive to examiners' signal that you are too lengthy. If there are no significant features in, for example, the past medical and family histories, just say so rather than go through a list of negatives.

You *must* rehearse presenting the abdominal findings in logical order again and again. An example is as follows:

> On examination, there are striae and a previous caesarean section scar. The fundus is at the level of the xiphisternum, and the fundal height is 36 cm, which is compatible with 36 weeks gestation. There appears on palpation to be a normal amount of amniotic fluid. The lie is longitudinal and the presentation cephalic; the head is engaged with one-fifth palpable. The fetal back is palpable on the left side, and the fetal heart is heard at a rate of 140 beats per minute.

A fluent presentation of such findings gives the examiners a good impression.

Routine antenatal investigations

N.B. Antenatal investigations vary amongst hospitals. The following is only one example, but gives a rough idea of the investigations to be carried out.

BOOKING (ABOUT 10 WEEKS)

Blood tests

- full blood count – check haemoglobin and MCV
- blood group (ABO and rhesus) and atypical antibody screen
- sickle cell screen for Negroes, haemoglobin electrophoresis if Asian (if these have not previously been performed
- rubella antibody screen – some centres perform the whole TORCHS screen (toxoplasma, rubella, cytomegalovirus, hepatitis B and syphilis) but most just screen for rubella unless there are any indications to the contrary

Urine

- test for glucose
- microscopy, culture and sensitivity

16 WEEKS

- Alphafetoprotein test for neural tube defect screening. If the result is positive, consider high-resolution ultrasound scanning or amniocentesis to measure the alphafetoprotein level.
- Routine ultrasound examination to determine the length of gestation, detect multiple pregnancy and detect major structural abnormalities.

Extra test

All mothers over 40 years of age, and some between 35 and 40, may need screening by amniocentesis for chromosomal abnormalities, especially for Down's syndrome. Alternatively, a triple test may be performed, to be followed by amniocentesis if positive.

SUBSEQUENT VISITS

The exact schedule varies, depending on the obstetrician and the support by the local GP. It is usually every 4 weeks until 32 weeks gestation, every 2 weeks until 36 weeks and then weekly until delivery.

Check haemoglobin and atypical antibody levels again at 32 weeks if the mother is rhesus negative.

At each visit (in addition to the usual clinical examinations) record the following:

- weight
- abdominal examination
- blood pressure
- urine test results (protein, glucose)
- ultrasound results if there are concerns about growth

Anaemia in pregnancy

This is diagnosed by a haemoglobin level of less than 10 g/dL.

HISTORY

- symptoms – tires easily
- predisposing factors:
  - poor diet
  - vomiting in pregnancy
  - many recent pregnancies
  - not taking iron and folic acid supplements

EXAMINATION

There are usually few signs except pallor of the conjunctivae.

INVESTIGATIONS

- haemoglobin level
- blood film and MCV – microcytosis and low MCV suggests iron deficiency, macrocytosis and high MCV suggests folate deficiency
- reticulocytes – high levels suggest that the patient is responding to treatment
- ferritin (or iron) level
- vitamin B_{12} and folate levels
- sickle cell screen (if Negro), haemoglobin electrophoresis (if Asian)

TREATMENT (assuming iron deficiency)

- Haemoglobin level >8 g/dL – ensure compliance, use 'double iron'. If the patient is not tolerating this, consider intramuscular injec-

tion (six injections on alternate days).
- Haemoglobin level <8 g/dL – before 35 weeks, admit and treat with intramuscular injections and observe the response. After 35 weeks, admit for transfusion.

Rhesus incompatibility

Box 5.2. Risk of rhesus incompatibility

Who is at risk?
- mother is rhesus negative and
- father is rhesus positive and
- baby is rhesus positive

Especially
- if mother has been sensitized to antigen by transfusion
- amniocentesis
- abortion
- delivery involving a rhesus positive baby and Anti-D has not been given

---

Box 5.3. Detection and management of rhesus incompatibility

Detection
- check rhesus blood group at booking
- check antibody level frequently
- carry out amniocentesis for optical density if high

Management
- intrauterine transfusion if severe
- consider early delivery
- phototherapy or exchange transfusion of the baby after delivery

---

Pregnancy-induced hypertension (pre-eclampsia)

HYPERTENSION IN PREGNANCY

- blood pressure of 140/90 or over on two occasions more than 4 hours apart, *or*
- an increase of 30mmHg (systolic) or 20mmHg (diastolic) over the booking blood pressure

Hypertension may be:

- pregnancy-induced hypertension (PIH) – if hypertension occurs for the first time after 20 weeks gestation
- pregnancy-associated hypertension (PAH) – if hypertension first occurs before 20 weeks gestation or before conception
- a mixture of PIH and PAH

Box 5.4. Cardinal signs of pre-eclampsia

- hypertension
- proteinuria

Box 5.5. History and signs of pre-eclampsia

History to elicit
- headache, especially frontal and occipital, and in the morning
- visual disturbance
- epigastric or hypochondrial pain
- jittery (fits if is severe, eclampsia)

Physical signs
- increase in blood pressure
- hyperreflexia
- clonus
- papilloedema, haemorrhages in fundi

Box 5.6. Investigations and management of pre-eclampsia

Investigations
- full blood count, clotting, U&E, uric acid level
- creatinine clearance, amount of protein in urine
- fetal well-being – CTG, ultrasound, Doppler measurement

Management
- bed rest
- ? early delivery
- ? antihypertensive – hydralazine or labetalol
- ? anticonvulsant – diazepam

Antepartum haemorrhage

Definition – bleeding from the genital tract after 24 weeks (previously 28) of pregnancy but before the onset of labour.

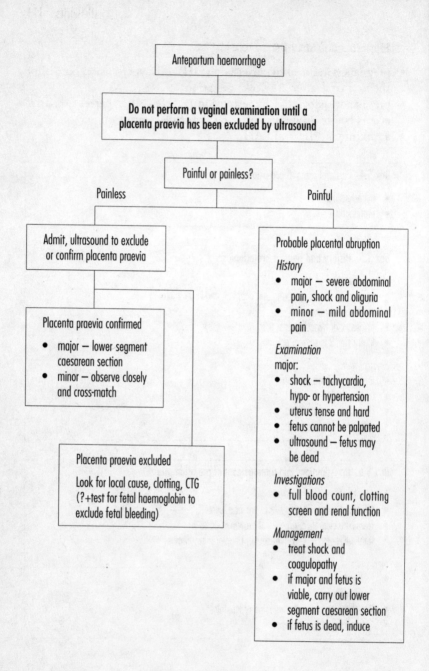

```
                    ┌──────────────────────────┐
                    │  Antepartum haemorrhage  │
                    └──────────────────────────┘
         ┌────────────────────────────────────────────────┐
         │  Do not perform a vaginal examination until a   │
         │  placenta praevia has been excluded by ultrasound│
         └────────────────────────────────────────────────┘
                    ┌──────────────────────────┐
                    │   Painful or painless?   │
                    └──────────────────────────┘
     Painless                                    Painful
```

Painless

Admit, ultrasound to exclude or confirm placenta praevia

Placenta praevia confirmed
- major — lower segment caesarean section
- minor — observe closely and cross-match

Placenta praevia excluded

Look for local cause, clotting, CTG (?+test for fetal haemoglobin to exclude fetal bleeding)

Painful

Probable placental abruption

History
- major — severe abdominal pain, shock and oliguria
- minor — mild abdominal pain

Examination
major:
- shock — tachycardia, hypo- or hypertension
- uterus tense and hard
- fetus cannot be palpated
- ultrasound — fetus may be dead

Investigations
- full blood count, clotting screen and renal function

Management
- treat shock and coagulopathy
- if major and fetus is viable, carry out lower segment caesarean section
- if fetus is dead, induce

5.1. Approach to antepartum haemorrhage

Established diabetes and pregnancy

Box 5.7. Effect of diabetes on pregnancy

Increased incidence of:
- abortion in first trimester
- intrauterine death
- pre-eclampsia
- polyhydramnios
- obstructed labour due to large-sized baby
- congenital abnormality (e.g. congenital heart disease)
- preterm delivery

Box 5.8. Effect of pregnancy on diabetes

- insulin requirements increase during pregnancy and suddenly decrease after delivery;
- may make proliferative retinopathy worse.

Box 5.9. Specific investigations for and management of diabetes in pregnancy

Investigations
- BM stix should be monitored frequently (three times a day)
- HbA1c level to confirm good control
- detailed ultrasound at 16 weeks for structural abnormality
- detailed cardiac ultrasound at 22 weeks for congenital heart disease
- review fetal growth by regular ultrasound (frequency depends on progress)

Management
- aim to avoid hyperglycaemia (BM about 4–9 mmol/L)
- teamwork with diabetic nurse and possibly general physicians
- planned induction of labour after 38 weeks (to minimize risk of obstructed labour)
- during labour – intravenous glucose and insulin infusion; possibly an epidural
- prevent prolonged labour (use syntocinon if necessary)

Labour

- first stage – from onset of regular contractions to full dilatation of the cervix
- second stage – from full dilatation of the cervix to the delivery of the anterior shoulder
- third stage – from delivery of the baby's anterior shoulder to delivery of the placenta

OPTIONS OF PAIN RELIEF IN LABOUR

- inhalational analgesia – e.g. Entonox (50 per cent nitrous oxide, 50 per cent oxygen)
- intramuscular pethidine
- epidural – especially in hypertension; anticipated prolonged labour, forceps delivery or caesarean section (e.g. a breech presentation), with multiple pregnancy or with severe pain in a primigravida
- pudendal block if forceps are necessary
- transcutaneous nerve stimulation – efficacy equivocal

MONITORING OF FETAL WELL-BEING BEFORE LABOUR

- kick chart – for reduced fetal movement
- routine ultrasound – for oligohydramnios and asymmetrical intrauterine growth retardation (rise in head/abdominal circumference ratio)
- unstressed CTGs – for poor beat-to-beat variation, lack of baseline variation and decelerations
- Doppler placental blood flow

SIGNS OF DISTRESS DURING LABOUR

- meconium-stained liquor
- CTG (preferably via a fetal scalp electrode):
  - bradycardia (rate less than 120)
  - tachycardia (rate more than 160)
  - lack of beat-to-beat variation
  - lack of baseline variation
  - decelerations other than pure type 1 (type 1 = deceleration only with contractions, quick recovery)
- fetal blood sampling (if CTG is abnormal):
  - pH <7.2 requires immediate delivery
  - pH 7.2–7.3 = repeat

INDICATIONS FOR FORCEPS DELIVERY

- elective:
  - maternal: hypertension, cardiac disease
  - fetal: prematurity, breech (delivery of head)
- fetal distress in second stage of labour
- delay in second stage of labour (due to poor maternal effort or poor contraction)

INDICATIONS FOR CAESAREAN SECTION

- elective:
  - two previous caesarean sections
  - cephalopelvic disproportion
  - severe pre-eclampsia
  - placenta praevia
  - placental insufficiency
  - active herpes simplex infection (now rare)
  - possible caesarean section or trial of labour:
    breach presentation in a primigravida
    one previous caesarean section and one other minor indication
- emergency:
  - fetal distress in first stage
  - abnormal lie or presentation
  - cord prolapse

FACTORS INCREASING RISK OF PERINATAL MORTALITY

- general maternal factors:
  - age >35 years
  - primigravida or parity >3
  - maternal height less than 150 cm (risk of cephalopelvic dispro-
    portion)
- past obstetric history:
  - premature labour
  - previous caesarean section(s)
  - placental abruption
  - recurrent abortions
  - intrauterine or perinatal death
  - fetal congenital abnormalities
- present pregnancy:
  - hypertension
  - diabetes
  - antepartum haemorrhage
  - multiple pregnancy
  - premature labour or rupture of membranes
  - malpresentation
  - intrauterine growth retardation

Example of an obstetric long case

HISTORY

Date: 5 June 1995

Personal information

Name:	Alison Hope	Age:	23
Marital status:	Married	Ethnicity:	English
Occupation:	Shop manager		

History of present pregnancy

Planned/unplanned: Planned
Contraception before pregnancy: Nil in last year, Marvelon previously
Usual period: K = 6/28
LMP: 18 September 1994   Gestation by dates 37 weeks/ultrasound 37 weeks
EDD: 25 June 1995

Antenatal care:
Booked at 12 weeks, given iron/folate supplements. Booking BP 100/60.
Usual investigation at 16 weeks, including AFP and ultrasound, normal.
Seen at 24 weeks, no problems noted. Followed up every 4 weeks until 32 weeks, then every 2 weeks until 36 weeks. Rhesus antibody not detected at 16, 28 or 32 weeks.

Presenting problems:
Routine antenatal check-up by GP 4 weeks ago – BP 140/100. Repeated as 140/95. No symptoms – no headache, abdominal pain, vomiting or visual disturbance.
Urine test by GP – protein ++.
Therefore referred to hospital.

Feeding plan: breast feeding

Past obstetric history

Year	Gestation	Antenatal	Intrapartum mode of delivery	Outcome, birthweight	Sex	Postnatal, feeding
1992	40	Nil significant	Normal vaginal	Livebirth, 3.1 kg	M	Nil significant Breast feeding Anti-D given

Past gynaecological history

Nil of note.
Last cervical smear 1993 – negative.

Past medical history

Tonsillectomy aged 5. Nil else.

Blood group: A negative   Rubella status: Immune
                                                 (by immunization).

Drugs (present and before pregnancy), allergies

Nil.

Family history

Twins: Nil.
Diabetes: Nil.
Others: Mother had psoriasis.

Social history

Smoking: 20 cigarettes per day, stopped 6 months before conception.
Alcohol: Socially only, 8 units per week, stopped 6 months before conception.
Illicit drugs: Nil.
Accommodation: Lives with husband and son in two-bedroomed terraced house.
No. of children at home: One (3-year-old boy).
Social support: Nil required.
Financial: No worries – husband bank manager.

Direct questioning

Nil significant, apart from mild backache in the past 2 months.

PHYSICAL EXAMINATION

General

Height: 170 cm   Weight: 90.4 kg
Anaemia: Not clinically anaemic.

CVS

Pulse: 65/minute.
BP: 130/90   JVP at angle of sternum.
Oedema: Mild oedema especially of face and fingers.
Heart sounds: Normal.

RS
Normal.

Abdomen
Inspection
Fundal height: At xiphisternum, 36 cm

Palpation and auscultation
No tenderness.
Lie: Longitudinal.
Presentation: Cephalic.
Fifths palpable: 2/5.
Back of fetus: On left.
Fetal heart: Heard.   Rate: 140/minute.

CNS
Reflexes normal, no clonus. Fundi normal with no haemorrhages.

Vaginal examination [not to be carried out in exams]
Not done.

Urine
Protein ++.

SUMMARY

A 23-year-old married English shop manager, gravida 2, para 1, now 37 weeks by dates and ultrasound who had uneventful care until 4 days ago when she had a raised BP of 140/100 and proteinuria. She was totally asymptomatic, and her reflexes and fundi normal. She was thought to have mild pre-eclampsia and was admitted for bed rest; the BP has now settled to 130/90.

[You may then be asked to present the abdominal findings about the criteria for admission of patients with pregnancy-induced hypertension and about the possible investigations and management of this patient.]

6
Gynaecology

General advice for long cases

In the finals exam, gynaecology is usually assessed by only one 'long case'. In some clinical schools, there are separate obstetrics and gynaecology exams, whereas in others, there is a combined exam in which the long case may either be obstetrics or gynaecology.

The usual time allowed for interviewing patients in gynaecology varies between clinical schools, but is usually about 30 minutes – less than that allowed for medicine or surgery. It is important to be comprehensive in the sections of the history and examination that are especially relevant (e.g. menstrual history) but not to spend too much time on other less relevant sections. The following list looks lengthy, but, in fact, it can be completed quite easily in 30 minutes.

It is probably even more important in gynaecology to be considerate and empathic to the patient as intimate personal questions need to asked in the history.

HISTORY (20 MINUTES)

Personal details
- name
- age
- marital status
- occupation

Presenting complaints
A list of the symptoms that the patient describes, e.g. painful periods, pelvic pain.

History of presenting complaint(s)
Enquire about details of the symptoms, for example:

- When did the symptoms start?
- Were they continuous or intermittent?
- How severe were the symptoms?

Always ask about associated symptoms, if relevant, of:

- vaginal discharge – colour, smell and amount
- period pain or pelvic pain
- pain on intercourse (dyspareunia)
- abdominal pain
- menstruation history (*see* below)
- possible genital prolapse
- urinary and bowel symptoms if there is a history of suggesting prolapse

Menstruation history

- age at menarche – the average age is 12 years; it is abnormal if outside the range 9–16 years
- usual menstrual cycle:
  - usual length of menstrual cycle (i.e. time between the first day of one period and the first day of the next period)
  - usual duration of a period
  - record the answer in the form 'K = 7/28'
  - if irregular, write down the longest and shortest length of menstrual cycle and duration of a period, for example, K = 3–7/ 24–30
- amount of bleeding:
  - if abnormally heavy, note down the number of tampons or towels used, whether there are any clots and the colour of the blood
  - ask about mid-cycle spotting
- date of LMP
- date of menopause (if relevant)

Date of last cervical smear

Past medical history

Only note down any chronic illnesses that are relevant or may influence anaesthetic requirements if surgery is needed (e.g. diabetes, congenital heart disease, bowel surgery or urological surgery).

Past obstetric and gynaecological history

Note down for each pregnancy:

- the year
- whether there were any major antenatal, perinatal or postnatal problems, including episiotomies
- the mode of delivery (normal vaginal, forceps, Ventouse or caesarean section)

- still birth or livebirth, gender of baby
- miscarriage or termination, the year and the gestation

Note down any previous gynaecological problems or surgical procedures undertaken (e.g. D&C).

Contraception used

Note the contraception used currently and in the past, and the reasons for the choice.

For menopausal patients, ask about the use of hormone replacement therapy (HRT).

Family and social history

Check any family history of breast or gynaecological malignancies.

Note who is living with the patient, the current living accommodation and current occupation.

Sexual history

Enquire into if it is relevant (e.g. if the presenting complaint is infertility or a request for termination).

PHYSICAL EXAMINATION (10 minutes)

General

Look for anaemia and hirsuitism.

Cardiovascular system

Note pulse rate and blood pressure. If there is no previous history of heart disease, auscultation of the heart for murmurs is sufficient.

Respiratory system

If there is no previous history of respiratory disease, a quick assessment of the respiratory rate and auscultation are sufficient.

Abdomen

This is the most important part of the physical examination you may carry out in the exam.

- *Inspect* for scars, striae, masses and distension.
- *Palpate* for masses, tenderness and the liver, spleen and kidneys. If a mass is palpable, decide whether it is the bladder by percussion. Determine its size, its consistency, whether the edges are smooth or irregular and its mobility.

- *Percuss* to outline the extent of a mass, to detect the bladder or to detect free fluid in the peritoneal cavity (dull in the flanks, resonant centrally).
- *Auscultate* bowel sounds if distension due to obstruction or ileus is suspected.

Breast examination

Check prior to the exam whether you are expected to perform this before you see the examiner. If you are not, always mention that you would in practice perform examination of the breast.

Breast examination should be performed systematically. Inspect for underlying endocrine changes (e.g. pigmentation or galactorrhoea), and palpate with the flat of the hand in each of the four quadrants for the presence of tumour.

Pelvic examination

You are *not* required to perform pelvic examination and are unlikely to be asked to perform it when the examiners arrive. However, you may be asked the technique of speculum and digital pelvic examination and the technique of taking a cervical smear.

Speculum examination

This should be performed before the digital examination.

Start with inspecting the external genitalia: vulva, labia, clitoris and urethral meatus.

A Cuscoe's (bivalve) speculum is the most commonly used. Fully insert the instrument (closed) into the vagina before opening the blades. Direct a light to allow the vaginal walls and the cervix to be seen. Look for vaginal discharge and any abnormalities of the cervical epithelium.

A cervical smear is usually taken using an Ayre's spatula, gently scraping on the epithelial surface (squamocolumnar junction) of the cervix, and applying the scrapings to a labelled glass slide, which is placed in preservative fluid.

A Sim's speculum is best used if genital prolapse is suspected, examination should be performed when the subject is in the lateral semi-prone position.

Digital examination

In bimanual examination, put lubricant on the right-hand glove and put the left hand on the abdomen to push the pelvic organs on to the right hand.

Look for:

- the position of the uterus — anteverted or retroverted (10 per cent of all normal woman have a retroverted uterus, but this is not significant as long as this is mobile)
- the size of uterus
- the consistency of uterus
- whether any mass is noted

Palpate the pouch of Douglas posteriorly and the fornices laterally for nodules or masses.

PRESENTATION

You should always prepare a short case summary of at most two sentences as the examiner may ask for it at the beginning. In any case, you need a summary at the end of the presentation. For example:

> Mrs X is a 24-year-old married teacher with two previous missed abortions 2 and 3 years ago, who has now presented with a 2-day history of lower abdominal pain and fresh vaginal bleeding after 8 weeks of amenorrhoea. This may be a case of inevitable abortion or, less likely, ectopic pregnancy.

You should present the history of the presenting complaint(s) succinctly, with important relevant negatives. Menstrual history, last cervical smear and contraception are important. For the rest of the history, you can state, 'There is nothing significant in the past medical history or family history' if this is the case. Similarly, in the physical examination, you should always mention the clinical presence or absence of anaemia if there is a history of heavy periods, and the examination findings of the abdomen need to be detailed. However, you can state, 'There is nothing significantly abnormal in the cardiovascular and respiratory system' if this is the case.

Abortion

This is defined as expulsion of the conceptus from the uterus before the 24th (previously 28th) week of gestation. (N.B. There is a need to exclude ectopic pregnancy first; suspicion is aroused by a positive beta-HCG with no fetus in uterus.)

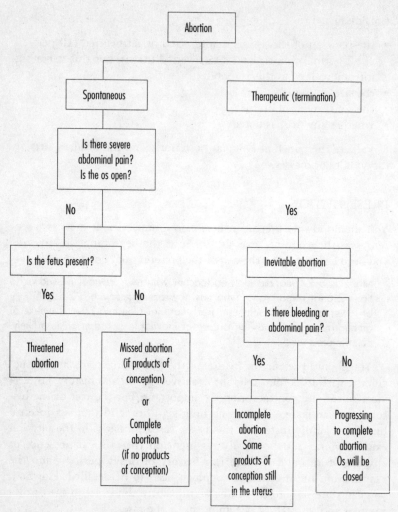

6.1 Approach to abortion

THERAPEUTIC ABORTION (TERMINATION)

Termination may be carried out if two medical practitioners (usually, but not necessarily, the GP and consultant gynaecologist) are of the opinion, and sign the relevant form, that at least one of the following applies.

- (If the pregnancy has not exceeded 24 weeks) Continuing the pregnancy would involve risk, greater than if the pregnancy were terminated, of:

- injury to the physical or mental health of the mother; or
- injury to the physical or mental health of any existing children of her family.
- Termination is necessary to prevent grave permanent injury to the physical or mental health of the pregnant mother.
- Continuing the pregnancy would involve risk to the life of the pregnant mother, greater than if the pregnancy were terminated.
- There is substantial risk that if the child were born, it would suffer from such physical or mental abnormalities as to be seriously handicapped.

Abnormal uterine bleeding

TERMS

- poly-   cycle occurring more often than 28 days
- -rhagia   excessive in amount
- metor-   occurs irregularly

MOST COMMON CAUSES

These vary according to age.

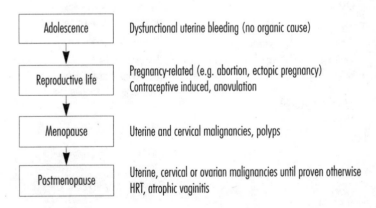

Adolescence	Dysfunctional uterine bleeding (no organic cause)
Reproductive life	Pregnancy-related (e.g. abortion, ectopic pregnancy) Contraceptive induced, anovulation
Menopause	Uterine and cervical malignancies, polyps
Postmenopause	Uterine, cervical or ovarian malignancies until proven otherwise HRT, atrophic vaginitis

ORGANIC CAUSES OF ABNORMAL BLEEDING

- *general* – blood coagulation disorder (e.g. low platelet count, Von Willebrand's disease); hyper- or hypothyroidism
- *ovarian* – tumours, follicular cysts: increased oestrogen
- *fallopian tube* – ectopic pregnancy, salpingitis

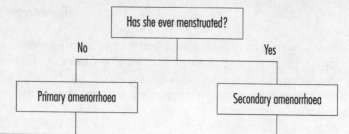

Has she ever menstruated?

No → **Primary amenorrhoea**

Yes → **Secondary amenorrhoea**

Primary amenorrhoea

- *Constitutional delay of menarche*
  Ask for a family history of similar delay

- *Turner's syndrome*
  Look for webbed neck, increased carrying angle and short stature

- *Cryptomenorrhoea* (e.g. imperforate hymen
  Ask for a history of cyclical pain at ovulation

- *Look for breast development*
  If present, suggest:
  − rare hypothalamic causes, (e.g. Kallman syndrome)
  − pituitary causes (e.g. tumour)
  − uterine causes (e.g. congenital absence)

  If absent, suggest:
  − ovarian causes (e.g. Turner's syndrome, gonadal dysgenesis)
  − testicular feminization
  − adrenal causes (e.g. mild adrenal hyperplasia)

Secondary amenorrhoea

- *Pregnancy*
  Ask for other symptoms of pregnancy, suggest a pregnancy test

- *Hypothalamic causes*
  Ask for stress or emotional upset
  Weight loss − ?anorexia nervosa

- *Drug induced*
  ask for contraceptive usage (progesterone-only pill), digoxin, phenothiazines give rise to increased prolactin

- *Pituitary causes*
  Especially prolactin-secreting tumour, which causes increase in prolactin levels
  Ask for headache and visual symptoms; check visual field and fundi for optic atrophy

- *Polycystic ovaries*
  Ask for hirsuitism and deepening of voice; suggest measuring FSH:LH ratio (>3)

- *Premature ovarian failure*

- *Uterine synechiae or endometrium ablation*
  Ask for a history of past gynaecological surgery

6.2 Approach to amenorrhoea

- *uterine* – fibroids, polyps, carcinoma, adenomyosis, pregnancy related (e.g. incomplete abortion or hydatiform mole)
- *cervical* – polyps, carcinoma and cervicitis
- *vagina* – atrophic vaginitis, foreign body

Amenorrhoea (Fig. 6.2)

Dysmenorrhoea

This is defined as pelvic pain occurring about the time of menstruation that is severe enough to interfere with the work and life of the subject.

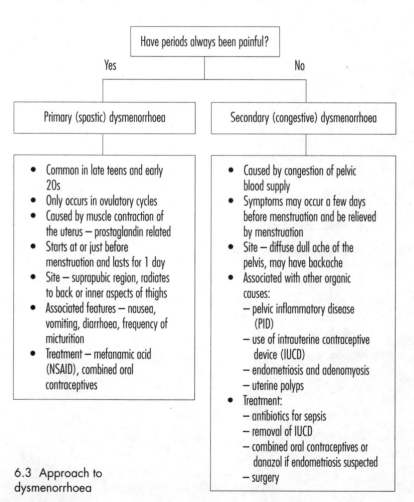

Have periods always been painful?

Yes → Primary (spastic) dysmenorrhoea

No → Secondary (congestive) dysmenorrhoea

Primary (spastic) dysmenorrhoea
- Common in late teens and early 20s
- Only occurs in ovulatory cycles
- Caused by muscle contraction of the uterus – prostaglandin related
- Starts at or just before menstruation and lasts for 1 day
- Site – suprapubic region, radiates to back or inner aspects of thighs
- Associated features – nausea, vomiting, diarrhoea, frequency of micturition
- Treatment – mefanamic acid (NSAID), combined oral contraceptives

Secondary (congestive) dysmenorrhoea
- Caused by congestion of pelvic blood supply
- Symptoms may occur a few days before menstruation and be relieved by menstruation
- Site – diffuse dull ache of the pelvis, may have backache
- Associated with other organic causes:
  - pelvic inflammatory disease (PID)
  - use of intrauterine contraceptive device (IUCD)
  - endometriosis and adenomyosis
  - uterine polyps
- Treatment:
  - antibiotics for sepsis
  - removal of IUCD
  - combined oral contraceptives or danazol if endometriosis suspected
  - surgery

6.3 Approach to dysmenorrhoea

Vaginal discharge

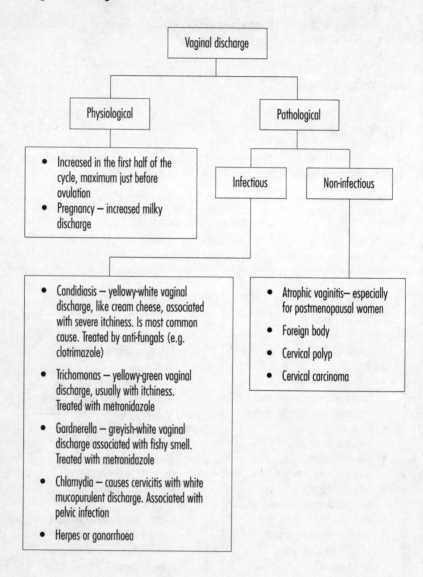

6.4 Approach to vaginal discharge

Infertility

HISTORY

Both partners

Details of intercourse – frequency, problems encountered, length of time not using contraceptives without pregnancy being achieved.
    Also note past contraceptive usage.

Male partner

- past medical history of:
    - undescended testis
    - mumps in adulthood
    - testicular tumour
    - malignant disease, use of chemotherapy and use of radiotherapy
    - sexually transmitted disease (e.g. gonorrhoea)
- social history of alcohol abuse
- sexual problems – impotence or premature ejaculation
- any sperm counts performed

Female partner

- present history of:
    - menstrual cycle
    - signs of ovulation (e.g. temperature chart or cyclical change of cervical mucus)
    - use of drugs causing hyperprolactinaemia (e.g. phenothiazines)
    - galactorrhoea
- past history of:
    - pelvic inflammatory disease
    - endometriosis
    - ectopic pregnancy
    - use of IUCD or injectable contraceptives
    - gynaecological operations (e.g. D&C)

INVESTIGATIONS

- male – sperm count after 3 days abstinence from intercourse; repeat if abnormal
- female:
    - test for ovulation (e.g. temperature chart, cervical mucus and endometrial biopsy)
    - hormone levels (e.g. prolactin, thyroid function, FSH and LH)

　　　– hysterosalpingogram and/or laparoscopy dye test for tubal
　　　patency
* both partners – postcoital test

Gynaecological cancers

Table 6.1. Gynaecological cancers

	Cervical	Uterine	Ovarian
Risk factors	Early age of coitus Promiscuity Human papillomavirus Herpes simplex infection Does not attend routine 　screening Peak age 40	Nulliparity Unopposed oestrogen 　therapy Peak age 60	?Nulliparity Peak age 50–60
Symptoms	Asymptomatic in early 　stages Abnormal smear *Abnormal bleeding* Postcoital bleeding Intermenstrual bleeding Postmenopausal bleeding *Late symptoms* Pain Discharge	Postmenopausal bleeding	Abdominal distension Abdominal pain
Signs	Lesion seen in cervix on 　speculum examination	Bulky uterus May be absent	Signs of ascites Abdominal mass Adnexal mass ?Swollen leg
Further investigations	Colposcopy Cone biopsy	Endometrial biopsy Ultrasound of uterus	Urea Tumour marker Chest X-ray Ultrasound Intravenous 　pyelography CT scan Laparotomy

Contraception

Table 6.2. Types of contraception

Type	How administered	Advantages	Disadvantages
Natural	*Calendar* Unsafe period – begins on day [length of longest cycle -18] ends on day [length of shortest cycle -10] *Symptomothermal* Temperature chart or cervical mucus Safe period – 3 days after ovulation	No side-effectives Costs nothing	High failure rate High motivation needed
Condom	Barrier method by male	Cheap Protects against sexually transmitted diseases Medical supervision not needed No side-effects	Reduces spontaneity Correct use essential
Cap/diaphragm with spermicide	Barrier method by female Spermicide must be applied within 2 hours before intercourse Must leave in place for 6 hours after intercourse	No side-effects Spontaneity preserved	Initial fitting by professional Motivation essential High risk rate for young
'The pill' (combined oral contraceptive; COC)	One tablet daily for 21 days followed by 7 pill-free days Effective immediately if started on day 1 of cycle (on day 15 if begun at any other time of cycle)	Highly effective Safe if closely monitored Reduction in: – dysmenorrhoea – irregular, heavy periods – endometriosis – premenstrual syndrome – fibrocystic breast disease – ovarian cysts/carcinoma	Extra precautions needed if vomiting or diarrhoea or if antibiotics are given Motivation important Increased risk of myocardial infarct, venous thrombo-embolism and fluid retention
'Mini-pill' (progesterone-only pill)	One tablet daily continuously Must be taken within same 3 hours on each day Effective from day 15	Useful: – in breast feeding – in older women – if troublesome oestrogenic side-effects from COC	High failure in young women Needs to be taken accurately Side-effects – irregular periods or amenorrhoea, increased risk of ectopic pregnancy

Table 6.2 (continued)

Type	How administered	Advantages	Disadvantages
Injectables	Intramuscular injection every 12 (Depro-provera) or 8 (Noristerat) weeks	Useful: – with rubella vaccine – postvasectomy – in developing countries – if other methods are unsuitable	May reduce fertility for >1 year Irregular bleeding Weight gain
IUCD ('the coil')	Inserted by doctors May need change every few years depending on type	No problem with forgetting Lasts for long time Relatively effective Reversible	Nulliparous unsuitable Increased risk of: – pelvic infection – heavy, irregular bleeding – ectopic pregnancy – expulsion and perforation
Subcutaneous implant (Norplant)	To be inserted only by trained doctors (introduced in UK 1992)	No problem with forgetting Lasts for long time Reversible (by removal) No oestrogenic side-effects	Good insertion technique essential Irregular bleeding Relatively new
Sterilization (male)	Performed by surgeons Effective only with three negative sperm counts after operation	Effective No further action required	Irreversible Possibility of recanalization
Sterilization (female)	By laparoscopy (clips) or laparatomy	Effective No further action required	Irreversible Possibility of recanalization
Postcoital contraception			
'Morning after pill' (e.g. Shering PC4)	Within 72 hours of intercourse; two tablets followed by a further two tablets after 12 hours	99% effective	Causes nausea Ineffective if vomiting occurs
IUCD	To be inserted within 5 days of unprotected intercourse Remove after next period	100% effective	Side-effects of IUCD, as above

Genital (uterine) prolapse

CLASSIFICATION

> **Box 6.1. Classification of genital prolapse**
> - first degree — cervix descended to the introitus
> - second degree — cervix descended through the introitus
> - third degree — whole uterus descended through the introitus

HISTORY

History of presenting complaint(s)

- awareness of 'something coming down', especially when standing;
- low backache
- urinary symptoms — hesitancy, frequency, incomplete emptying, stress incontinence (leakage of urine on coughing), due to prolapse of the bladder: cystolcele
- difficulty emptying rectum (due to prolapse of rectum: 'rectocele')

Past history

- history of childbirth, especially by vaginal delivery with prolonged second stage or large babies
- history predisposing to increased intra-abdominal pressure (e.g. COAD, constipation or obesity)

Social history

Smoking predisposes to chronic cough.

PHYSICAL EXAMINATION

Abdomen

Look for an abdominal mass (giving rise to increased intra-abdominal pressure).

Pelvic examination (not required in finals exam)

- ask the subject to bear down, to assess the degree of prolapse
- ask the subject to cough, to demonstrate the presence or absence of stress incontinence
- use a Sims' speculum with the subject in left lateral position to assess the descent of the uterus and anterior and posterior vaginal walls

Example of a gynaecology long case

HISTORY

Personal details

Name:	Mary Smith	Age:	29
Marital status:	Married	Occupation:	Teacher

Presenting complaint(s)

Amenorrhoea.

History of presenting complaint(s)

Menarche aged 13, established regular periods K = 7/28 with normal amount of bleeding and no dysmenorrhoea.

Took Marvelon aged 22. Regular withdrawal bleeds, slightly later than normal periods.

Came off Marvelon 1 year 6 months ago, as she and her husband were planning a family. Since then, she has had no menstruation. She has no other symptoms. There has been no glactorrhoea, no visual disturbance and no history of weight loss in the last 18 months; no hirsuitism or voice changes. She has admitted to feeling quite stressed by her job.

Associated features:

- vaginal discharge: nil
- pelvic pain: nil
- dyspareunia: nil
- prolapse: nil
- abdominal pain: nil
- bowel and urinary symptoms [if relevant]: nil.

Menstruation history

- age of Menarche: 13
- usual period: K = 3/28 (when on Marvelon before) 18 months ago; no periods since then
- how heavy: N/A
- LMP: 18 months ago

Past obstetric history

No previous pregnancy.

Past gynaecological history

Nil of note.
Last cervical smear September 1994 – normal.

Past medical history

Mild asthma since childhood. Now well controlled on Ventolin inhaler prn only.
No other significant history.

Drug history

Ventolin inhaler 2 puffs prn (only needed once a week on average).

Allergies

Nil.

Family/social history

Mother (47) is a teacher, A&W; father (48) sailor, A&W. No siblings.
Married since aged 23, happy marriage. Husband aged 30, decorator.
Smokes 5 cigarettes per day; alcohol 2 pints weekends only.
Lives in own two-bedroomed, terraced house with husband.
Has been a teacher for the past 7 years. Two years ago, she was promoted to Deputy Head, which she found quite stressful, especially since the school attained grant-maintained status.

PHYSICAL EXAMINATION

General

Height: 165 cm. Weight 70 kg.
No anaemia. Thyroid not palpable; thyroid status euthymic. No hirsuitism. Voice normal.
Breasts and secondary sexual development: Normal.

CVS

Pulse: 90/minute
BP: 120/80
Rest of CVS normal.

RS

RR = 15/minute. No recession; chest clear.

Abdomen

No surgical scars, no distension, soft and non-tender, no masses palpable. No liver, spleen or kidneys palpable.

CNS

Fundi and visual fields appear normal.

Pelvic examination

[Do not attempt in finals exam] Not done.

SUMMARY/DIAGNOSIS

A 29-year-old married teacher who has had secondary amenorrhoea for 18 months after having taken combined oral contraceptives for 6 years. She admitted to stress over the past 2 years due to her job. Physical examination was unremarkable.

COMMENTS

This example is given to show that a gynaecological history is often quite short, with no physical findings found on examination. However, the examiners will discuss with you the relevant investigations and management.

It is now thought that if there are no periods after coming off the pill for 6 months, there is usually an underlying cause and 'post-pill amenorrhoea' is not a diagnosis in itself. The cause may have been present for many years but was not apparent as withdrawal bleeding was maintained by the pill.

Prolactin level, thyroid function and FSH/LH ratio need to be measured as a first line of investigation of the cause. Subsequent management may include induction of ovulation by clomiphene if the woman wants to become pregnant.

7
Psychiatry

General advice for long cases

In some clinical schools, there is a separate psychiatry finals exam. However, in most clinical schools, it is part of the medical finals, when the long case may be in general medicine, paediatrics or psychiatry. Psychiatry is usually examined by a long case, although candidates may rarely be asked to elicit certain features of mental state in the short cases.

Many candidates are nervous about having a psychiatry case. This may be due to many factors. First, they have the impression that psychiatry patients are not able to give a good history. While this may be true, the organizers of the finals exams usually do their best to make sure that the patients can give a coherent history. If not, you can always tell the examiner at the beginning of the presentation, and the examiners will be able to see for themselves when they interview the patient with you. Second, a longer social and personal history must be obtained, and the student has to perform a mental state examination. Third, students worry that they have spent much less time in psychiatry than in general medical attachments. Fourth, the diagnosis in psychiatry may not be clear cut. However, this is also true for many other specialties, and a list of differential diagnoses is acceptable.

The key to success in the psychiatry long case rests in developing a good approach to history taking and mental state examination (*see* Box 7.1).

Box 7.1. Approach to the psychiatric case

When you are interviewing the patient, you should ask yourself the following questions.

1. How would you describe the symptoms? (e.g. depression, delusions, hallucinations)
2. What is this due to? (e.g. organic pathology, schizophrenia, alcohol or drugs)
3. Why does it happen to this patient? (e.g. genetics – family history; social situation – high expressed emotions; psychological – bereavement)
4. Why does it present now? (e.g. withdrawal of social support, recent discontinuation of medication)

In your formulation, you should try, if possible, to give relevant points on each of these areas.

HISTORY (about 25 minutes)

Personal details

Name: Occupation:
Age: Inpatient/outpatient:
Marital status: (If inpatient) Informal or on Section:

Presenting complaint(s)

Give brief details of the symptoms and their duration, for example, 'a 2-week history of insomnia, hearing voices and a feeling of being persecuted by the devil'.

History of presenting complaint(s)

This should consist of:

- general circumstances in which the symptoms arise;
- elaboration of the symptoms above; for example, when he started to hear voices, whether the voices are outside or inside his head, whose voices they are, whether they speak in the second or third person, the content of the voices, what the patient thinks about the voices.

Important negatives need to be recorded. For example, for patients with depression, appetite, weight change, sleep patterns and diurnal variations must be recorded.

Past medical history

Do not try to be overdetailed. Try to concentrate on chronic illnesses and any history that may give rise to the present symptoms. Thyroid diseases, diabetes, epilepsy and neurological disorders are important.

Past psychiatric history

This needs to be taken in detail. Note for each episode:

- the year when the illness started
- brief symptoms
- the diagnosis
- whether the patient was treated as an outpatient or admitted
- the treatment given
- how long treatment was continued. If treatment has stopped, was this on medical advice or by the patient?

For example:

1990 – Hears devil talking about him. Diagnosed with schizophrenia, and was admitted compulsorily for 5 months, when a depot injection was given. Medication continued for 1 year afterwards, and was stopped on patient's refusal of it.

Medication

Any prescribed drugs, including depot injections.

Allergies

Family history

- parents' ages, occupations and histories of mental illness
- sibling's forenames, ages, occupation and histories of mental illness
- children's forenames, ages, occupations and histories of mental illness

If you are short of time, forenames can be omitted.

Social history

Illicit drugs, alcohol and smoking

This aspect of the history, especially illicit drugs and alcohol, is extremely important.

For illicit drug use, note the type(s) of drug, route(s) by which they are taken (sniffing, orally or intravenously), the amount, source and whether they are taken alone or in groups.

For alcohol, note the number of units consumed (*see* Table 7.4) and any signs of dependence (*see* Box 7.4), and use the CAGE questionnaire.

General

Note with whom the patient is living, current interests, hobbies and clubs and any support by professionals (e.g. community psychiatric nurses or social workers) or informal carers.

Take details of the conditions of the patient's living accommodation.

Personal history

(This can be considerably shortened if there is insufficient time.)

- birth history:
  - Was the patient premature?
  - Was it a normal delivery?
  - Were there any perinatal problems?

- developmental history – developmental milestones: Any childhood neurotic traits?
- childhood:
  - Was it a happy childhood?
  - How does the patient get on with parents and siblings?
  - Was/is there any sibling rivalry?
- schooling and further education:
  - place of primary and secondary schooling
  - Does the patient get on well with academic work, with teachers and with fellow students?
  - date of leaving school and qualifications obtained
  - details of further education, and qualifications obtained
- occupational history – list occupations, their dates and reasons for leaving them
- psychosexual history:
  - previous sexual relationships, the duration and quality of the relationships, and the reasons for their termination
  - dates of engagement, marriage and/or divorce
- forensic history – ask about any trouble with the police, any previous convictions and the year and outcome of the convictions. This is particularly important if there is a history of aggression or violence

Premorbid personality

Ask the patient what type of person he or she usually was before the illness, both from the patient's point of view and from that of others (e.g. relatives). Record this in phrases such as 'shy', 'extrovert', 'happy'. It must, however, be remembered that the description of the premorbid personality elicited from the patient may be inaccurate.

PHYSICAL EXAMINATION (about 10 minutes)

You will not have time to perform a full physical examination; look only for signs that are relevant to your case.

For example, in patients with anxiety, look for signs of thyrotoxicosis – tachycardia, sweating, tremor, hyperreflexia, etc. – and for signs of Grave's disease – the eye signs of lid retraction, lid lag and exophthalmos.

For patients on antipsychotic drugs, take the blood pressure and look for side-effects of tremor, rigidity, oro-facial dyskinesia, akathisia, etc.

For patients with unexplained psychiatric symptoms and suspected organic syndromes, you may have to carry out a full neurological examination, including fundal appearance, language abilities, construction abilities and testing for agnosias.

MENTAL STATE EXAMINATION (about 15 minutes)

This is essential in a psychiatric case. You can probably make comments under many of these headings after your history taking. Hence, although the list looks long, you can perform the whole mental state examination in about 15 minutes. Again, it is important to concentrate on the headings that are particularly relevant to your case.

Appearance and behaviour

- Is the manner of dress appropriate or is it odd? Are hygiene and self-care good?
- Is the patient sitting down calmly or agitated and pacing up and down the room; is he or she anxious?
- Is the posture normal or are there symptoms of catatonia?
- What is the quality of eye contact and rapport?
- Is the patient friendly or hostile?

Speech

If there is obvious abnormality in the speech, you should record a sample of the speech for illustration.

- Rate and quantity. Is the patient speaking faster than average (pressure of speech), or is the speech slower than expected (retarded speech)? Is speech spontaneous or only in answer to questions? Are the answers monosyllables, single words, phrases or sentences?
- Flow. Is the patient logical, is he or she jumping from one subject to another by rhyming or clang association (flight of ideas). Is he or she jumping from one subject to another without any association (derailment) or is he or she totally incoherent?
- Content. Note down any abnormalities in the content of the speech.

Mood

- Objectively. Does he or she appear elated or depressed, or does his or her mood vary from one moment to another (is it labile)?
- Subjectively. Does the patient feel happy or sad in him or herself? Are there any ideas of self-harm?

Note any biological symptoms such as weight loss, loss of appetite, loss of enjoyment (anhedonia) or sleep disturbance that you may have elicited in the history of presenting complaint(s).

- Affect. This relates to emotional state over a shorter period of time during the interview. Abnormalities include incongruity of affect (e.g. laughing while telling a sad story), or flattened or blunted affect (e.g. showing little emotion during the interview).

Thought

If the patient appears psychotic, ask directly about thought insertion, thought withdrawal and thought broadcasting, and passivity feelings.

Note down any delusions (false beliefs held in spite of evidence to the contrary, which are out of keeping with the patient's social and cultural setting).

Note down any thoughts of persecution, self-importance (grandiose), hopelessness or worthlessness, and ideas of reference (that the TV or newspaper, for example, is talking about the patient).

See also page 157 for assessing risk of suicide.

Ask about obsessive thought if there is any evidence of obsessive compulsive symptoms.

Perception

Ask about any hallucinations (perceptions without stimulis), which are usually auditory or visual; olfactory or tactile hallucinations are rare.

Note (if auditory) their frequency, whether they are outside or inside the head, how many voices there are, whose voices they are, whether they speak in the second or third person, their content and the patient's reaction.

Cognition

It is important to test for cognition if the patient appears confused or muddled; if not, this section may be shortened.

- orientation – in time, place and person (this may be obvious during the history-taking)
- attention and concentration – depending on the patient's educational background, ask him or her:
  - to count backwards from 20
  - to call out the months of the year backwards
  - to recite serial 7s
- memory:
  - short-term memory: ask the patient to repeat a 6 digit number to you immediately after you. If this is accurate, ask the patient to repeat it again 5 minutes later. Give the patient a name and

address, and ask for it 5 minutes later
- recent memory: ask for recent news and details of the patient's daily living
- remote memory: dates of World War I and II, name of previous Prime Minister, etc.

Insight

This is important, especially if the patient has a psychotic or dementing illness. Ask whether he regards him or herself as having an illness and, if so, whether the illness is physical or mental. For delusions, test how strong the delusions are (is it possible that this is not true?). Ask whether he/she feels he/she requires any treatment.

PRESENTATION (10 minutes)

Preparation

This includes final questions to the patient on any topic you wish to clarify, putting the notes in order and preparing your summary and a list of differential diagnoses.

Presentation

You should present your history, mental state examination and physical examination in full, unless you are told otherwise by the examiners. However, you should aim to present only the positive points and the important relevant negatives. For example, in a patient with schizophrenia, the facts that there was no thought withdrawal, thought broadcasting, etc., are important relevant negatives, while the fact that there is no obsessive thought is not. Watch non-verbal communications from the examiners that your presentation is too lengthy and adjust accordingly.

Summary

You should always be prepared to give a summary of no more than three sentences succinctly summarizing the gist of the case. The examiners may ask for this summary at the beginning of your presentation; otherwise, you should give it at the end.
   In your summary, include:

- patient's age
- marital status
- sex
- occupation
- brief presenting complaints, duration and precipitating factors

- past psychiatric history (if relevant)
- relevant past medical history (if any) that contributes to the present symptoms
- any points in the family, social or personal histories that positively contribute to the patient's present illness
- a brief summary of the mental state examination (if not included in 'presenting complaints' above)

Examples are:

Mrs X is a 36-year-old single teacher who has had three episodes of severe depression in the past 5 years and now presents with a 1-month history of low mood and feelings of hopelessness and worthlessness, with biological symptoms of depression, which has partially responded to a course of fluoxetine. The symptoms have been partly triggered by the recent death of her mother.

Mr Y is a 47-year-old unemployed gentleman who has since 1980 suffered from paranoid schizophrenia, requiring several compulsory admissions to hospital, the last being in September 1993. He presents with a 2-month history of insomnia, paranoid delusions, ideas of reference and auditory hallucinations in the third person with derogatory comments; the symptoms started 3 months after he stopped his depot injections. He had a strong family history of schizophrenia, and there has been high expressed emotion at home.

Differential diagnosis

You should give the most likely diagnosis first, followed by those that are less likely. However, you should consider your diagnosis in the following order.

1. Are the mental symptoms caused by an organic illness (e.g. thyrotoxicosis causing anxiety symptoms, hypercalcaemia causing confusion or infection causing delirium)?
2. Are the mental symptoms caused by drugs (prescribed or illicit) or alcohol (e.g. benzodiazepines causing confusion, alcohol withdrawal causing delirium tremens or amphetamine-induced psychosis)?
3. Is it a functional psychosis (schizophrenia or bipolar affective disorder)?
4. Is it an affective disorder (mania or depression)?
5. Is it an obsessive–compulsory disorder or other neurosis (e.g. generalized anxiety disorder or phobic anxiety disorder)?
6. Is it a personality disorder?

In general, if there is equal evidence for diagnosis in more than one category, the top category should take priority; for example, in a patient with both recent depression and phobic anxiety symptoms, the primary diagnosis should be depression.

Investigations

Investigations that you should consider in psychiatry include:

- full blood count – anaemia may cause lethargy, raised MCV may indicate alcohol abuse and raised WBC may indicate infection
- U&E – electrolyte imbalance (e.g. uraemia or hyponatraemia) may cause confusion
- liver function tests (including gamma-GT) – liver failure may cause encephalopathy, raised gamma-GT may indicate alcohol abuse
- thyroid function test – hyperthyroidism may mimic an anxiety disorder, while hypothyroidism may mimic depression. This is also important when prescribing lithium, which may cause either hyper- or hypothyroidism
- lithium level – mandatory if lithium is prescribed
- urinary drug screen – important in detecting mental symptoms induced by illicit drugs
- EEG – may indicate causes for organic psychosis (e.g. infection, metabolic disorder or brain tumour) or underlying temporal lobe epilepsy
- CAT scan – important to rule out intracranial pathology
- psychometric tests – to assess personality and general intelligence, or localize brain changes (e.g. to detect whether there are frontal and temporal or parietal abnormalities)

Organic causes of psychiatric disorders – delirium

The presence of symptoms in each of the following categories should alert you to look for organic (physical) causes of the mental symptoms (adapted from ICD-10 classification).

- impairment of consciousness and attention:
  - ranges from mild (clouding of consciousness) to severe (coma)
  - tested (in order of difficulty) by asking the patient to name the days of weeks forwards and backwards, to count backwards from 20 or to recite serial 7s
- disturbance of cognition or perception:
  - disorientated in time, place or person
  - impairment of registration and short-term memory (tested by

asking the patient to register and recall after 5 minutes a 5 or 6
digit number or an address)
- visual illusions or hallucinations
• psychomotor disturbances:
- under- or over-activity, or rapid shift from one to the other
- increased or reduced flow of speech
• disturbance of sleep wake cycle:
- insomnia
- day-time drowsiness
- nocturnal worsening of symptoms
- nightmares
• emotional disturbances (e.g. depression, anxiety, fear or irritability)

ORGANIC CAUSES OF PSYCHIATRIC SYMPTOMS

• infection (e.g. meningitis, encephalitis, pneumonia)
• metabolic (e.g. hypercalcaemia)
• vitamin deficiency (e.g. vitamin B_1 and B_{12} deficiencies)
• endocrine abnormalities (e.g. Cushing's syndrome, hyper- or
  hypothyroidism)
• carcinoma
• liver or renal failure
• intracranial pathology (e.g. tumour)
• drugs (prescribed or illicit, e.g. isoniazid, digoxin or ampheta-
  mines) or alcohol

Diagnosis of schizophrenia

According to ICD-10 guidelines, diagnosis requires a one-month history of the following:

One clear-cut or two less clear-cut symptoms from sections 1–4 below:

1. thought echo – hearing own thoughts aloud
   - thought insertion – experience of thoughts being put into the
     mind
   - thought withdrawal – experience of thoughts taken out of the
     mind
   - thought broadcasting – experience that others can read or hear
     his or her thought
2. delusions of control, influence or passivity
   - delusional perception – delusion arises suddenly and illogically
     from a certain perception, e.g. believing that one is chosen by

God when seeing the traffic lights turn from red to green
3. auditory hallucination giving a running commentary
   −auditory hallucination discussing the patient amongst themselves
   − auditory hallucination coming from some part of the body
4. − persistent delusions that are culturally inappropriate and completely impossible

Or symptoms from two of groups 5–9 below:

5. persistent visual, olfactory or tactile hallucinations, either associated with fleeting delusions or if they occur every day for weeks
6. incoherency or irrelevance of speech, or neologisms (new word invented by the patient to describe his or her unusual experience)
7. catatonic behaviour (e.g. excitement, unnatural posture, stupor or mutism)
8. 'negative' symptoms − apathy, poverty of speech, blunted or incongruous (inappropriate) affect and social withdrawal
9. significant change in the quality of personal behaviour (e.g. a loss of premorbid interest, idleness, and social withdrawal)

Findings from history and examination
(*see* Table 7.1)

Comparison of findings in mania/hypomania and depression
(*see* Table 7.2)

Assessing risk of suicide

The risk of suicide should be assessed in every patient. This is especially the case after an episode of deliberate self-harm.

Factors increasing risk of suicide after an episode of deliberate self-harm:

- present episode:
  − premeditated
  − intended actions with serious consequences
  − violent methods
  − suicide note
- past medical history:

Table 7.1. Comparison of findings in different types of schizophrenia

	Paranoid	Hebephrenic	Catatonic	Simple
History				
General	Most common	Usually starts between 15 and 25 years of age	Rare in developed countries	Uncommon, only diagnosed if lasts >1 year
History of presenting complaint(s)	Paranoid delusions Auditory hallucinations	Unpredictable, irresponsible behaviour Incoherent	Extremes of over-reactivity and stupor Unnatural postures	Insidious, progressive oddities of conduct, social withdrawl and decline, loss of initiative
Past psychiatric history		Past history of episodes of the same symptoms		
Family history		Family history of schizophrenia		
Social and personal history	Relatively stable	Quick social decline	Good between episodes	Gradual social decline
Mental state examination				
Appearance and behaviour	Suspicious	Grimaces, mannerisms, self-satisfied smile	Extremes of overactivity and stupor, unnatural postures	Withdrawn Self-neglect
Speech	Abnormalities not prominent	Rambling, incoherent	Uncommunicative	Poverty in quantity and content
Mood and effect	Relatively normal	Shallow and inappropriate		Blunted affect, lack of emotional response

Table 7.1 (continued)

	Paranoid	Hebephrenic	Catatonic	Simple
Thought	Paranoid delusions Passivity, other delusions	Prominent thought disorder with incoherence and marked derailment	Difficult to assess	Abnormalities not usually prominent
Perception	2nd person auditory hallucination giving commands or 3rd person auditory hallucinations	Abnormalities not usually prominent	Difficult to assess	Abnormalities not usually prominent
Cognition	Intact	May be affected in late stages	Difficult to assess	May be affected in late stages
Insight	Little insight during episodes	Little insight	Difficult to assess	Usually little insight
Prognosis	Relatively good	Poor development of negative rapid symptoms	Generally good in long term	Poor

Table 7.2. Comparison of mania/hypomania and depression

	Hypomania/mania	Depression
History		
History of presenting complaints	Elevation of mood Increased energy/activity Reduced sleep Overspending Increased sexual activity Risk-taking pursuits	Feels sad Loss of interest and enjoyment (anhedonia) Lethargy, tiredness Insomnia Reduced appetite or weight
Past psychiatric history	History of hypomania/depression	History of depression or hypomania and depression
Family history	History of bipolar affective disorder	History of depression or bipolar affective disorder
Social history	Recent increase in smoking and/or alcohol taking	More likely to be employed, divorced, widowed or single Alcohol abuse
Personal history		Death of mother at a young age
Mental state examination		
Appearance and behaviour	Talkative, overfamiliar Irritable, agitated Overactive, distractable	Signs of self-neglect Poor eye contact and rapport
Speech	Pressure of speech Flights of ideas Clang associations	Little spontaneous speech Retarded speech Nihilistic content
Mood and affect	Elevated or irritable mood	Low mood
Thought	Persecutory or grandiose thoughts	Worthlessness, guilty thoughts Hopelessness, suicidal thoughts
Perception	Second-person auditory hallucinations of grandiose content	Second-person auditory hallucinations, usually derogatory
Cognition	Intact, but test affected by distractability	Intact, but test affected by lack of motivation (pseudodementia)
Insight	Usually poor	May be present or absent

- chronic disability
- past psychiatric history:
  - past history of schizophrenia or depression
  - previous history of deliberate self-harm
  - borderline personality disorder
  - drug abuse
  - alcohol abuse
- family and social history:
  - family history of suicide or mental illness
  - single or divorced
  - living alone
  - unemployed
- mental state examination:
  - signs of severe depression, especially agitated depression
  - (lack of regret at suicide attempt)
  - feelings of hopelessness
  - ideas of suicide (N.B. One does *not* put ideas into the patient's mind by asking the questions. One can start with questions such as, 'Do you sometimes feel life is not worth living?' and progress to, 'Have you made any plans?', etc. For delusions, explore the reasons for suicide from the patient's point of view.)

Neurotic disorders

PHOBIC ANXIETY DISORDER

1 (a) *Psychological* symptoms of anxiety (apprehension and fear of object/situation, and secondary fear of dying, losing control, going mad, etc.).
  (b) *Autonomic* symptoms of anxiety (e.g. palpitation, dizziness, dry mouth, epigastric discomfort).
2. Anxiety is *restricted* to the feared object or situation (e.g. presence of animals for animal phobia; social situations in social phobia, and crowds, public places, travelling alone and travelling away from home in agoraphobia).
3. The patient *avoids* the feared object or situation.

GENERAL ANXIETY DISORDER

Anxiety is generalized and persistent, not restricted to or strongly predominated in any particular situation, and occurring at least several weeks at a time. Symptoms consist of:

- psychological complaints – worrying, difficulty in concentrating, feeling 'on edge'
- motor tension (e.g. fidgeting, tension headaches and not being able to relax)
- autonomic overactivity

PANIC DISORDER

Recurrent attacks of severe anxiety (panic) not restricted to any particular situations, which last for minutes or longer. Symptoms consist of:

- psychological complaints – particularly a fear of dying, losing control or going mad
- autonomic overactivity
- being relatively free of symptoms between attacks, although patients are often worried about another attack (anticipatory anxiety)

OBSESSIVE–COMPULSIVE DISORDER

There may be the following:

- obsessive thoughts:
  (a) thoughts or images repetitively enter the subject's mind
  (b) these ideas or images are unpleasant
  (c) they are recognized as the subject's own thoughts
  (d) the subject often unsuccessfully attempts to resist these thoughts
- compulsive acts:
  (a) stereotyped behaviours that are repeated over and over again (e.g. counting, cleaning or washing the hands)
  (b)–(d) above apply

Dementia

This is defined as a 6-month history of global deterioration in cognitive function, thinking and personality in clear consciousness sufficient to impair the personal activities of daily living.

HISTORY

- forgetfulness, irritability to learn new material
- change in personality (e.g. antisocial behaviour such as sexual disinhibition or shoplifting)

- loss of emotional control or sudden mood changes
- impaired judgement
- rigid routines

Late stages

- self-neglect
- nominal dysphasia
- disorientation and wandering
- incontinence of urine and faecies

MENTAL STATE EXAMINATION

- appearance and behaviour:
  - signs of self-neglect, disinhibition and mannerisms
  - agitation or apathy
- speech:
  - perseveration, dysphasia and syntactical errors
  - may become incoherent in late stages
- mood:
  - may be depressed, anxious or irritable
  - sudden unexplained mood changes
- thought:
  - poverty of thought
  - rigid concrete thought
  - may have paranoid delusions
- perception:
  - sometimes hallucinations
- cognition – impairment in all areas of intellectual functioning:
  - impairment of registration and recall (e.g. digit span), especially for recent events
  - impairment of concentration (e.g. days of week backwards)
  - impairment of language functions (e.g. poor comprehension, dysphagia and neologisms)
  - may have apraxias (e.g. inability to draw a clock face)
  - may have agnosias (e.g. inability to identify an object placed in the hand or, with the eyes closed, to identify which of his or her fingers is being touched)
- insight – usually lost in Alzheimer's disease, better preserved in the early stages of multi-infarct dementia

MOST COMMON CAUSES OF DEMENTIA

Table 7.3. Common causes of dementia

	Alzheimer's disease	Vascular dementia
Onset	Insidious	More abrupt
Deterioration	Slowly over several years	Stepwise deterioration
Associated features	Family history of Alzheimer's disease in those with onset at younger age	Increased blood pressure, carotid bruit, transient ischaemic attacks or cerebrovascular accidents, focal neurological signs
Clinical features		
Cognitive impairment	Global	Uneven
Personality	Affected early	Relatively well preserved
Judgement	Affected early	Relatively well preserved
Insight	Affected early	Relatively well preserved

Alcohol abuse

LEVELS OF CONSUMPTION

Table 7.4. Alcohol consumption (per week)

	Men	Women
Safe	<28 units	<21 units
Hazardous	28–49 units	21–35 units
Dangerous	>49 units	>35 units

ALCOHOL CONTENTS

Box 7.2. Alcohol contents

1 unit
= glass of table wine
= 1 (conventional) glass of sherry
= 1 (bar) measure of spirits
= a half pint of beer

CAGE QUESTIONNAIRE

Two positive replies out of four to the questions in Box 7.3 indicate problem drinking.

Box 7.3. CAGE questionnaire

- Have you ever felt you ought to cut down on your drinking?
- Have people annoyed you by criticizing your drinking?
- Have you ever felt guilty about you drinking?
- Have you ever had a drink first thing in the morning (an eye opener)?

PHYSICAL CONSEQUENCES OF ALCOHOL INTAKE

- gastrointestinal – oesophageal varices, oesophagitis, peptic ulcer, pancreatitis, stomach and oesophageal carcinoma
- liver – fatty liver, alcoholic hepatitis, cirrhosis, heptocellular carcinoma
- neurological – peripheral neuropathy, optic atrophy, myopathy, cerebellar degeneration, Wernicke's encephalopathy (clouding of consciousness, ocular palsy/nystagmus and peripheral neuropathy) and Korsakoff's syndrome (inability to form new memory, confabulation and peripheral neuropathy)
- other – anaemia, cardiomyopathy, increased rate of infection, especially tuberculosis, fetal alcohol syndrome in babies, increased risk of head injury

ALCOHOL DEPENDENCE

Box 7.4. Alcohol dependence

Indicated by three of the following:
- strong sense of *compulsion* to drink
- difficulty in *controlling* the level of drinking
- physiological *withdrawal* state, or use of alcohol to *relieve*/avoid withdrawal
- *tolerance*, with increasing intake of alcohol
- *neglect* of other interests
- *persistence* of drinking despite harmful effects

PSYCHIATRIC EFFECT OF ALCOHOL ABUSE

- withdrawal symptoms
- delirium tremens:
  - in patients with alcohol dependence
  - 2–4 days after total or partial withdrawal of alcohol
  - clouding of consciousness with disorientation, impairment of recent memory
  - severe agitation and restlessness, inattention, visual (and rarely auditory) hallucination and misinterpretation of stimuli, tremulousness, sweating, fever, tachycardia and dilatation of pupils
  - worse at night
  - needs emergency treatment in a medical ward
- Wernicke's and Korsakoff's syndrome (*see* above)
- alcohol hallucinosis – hearing insulting or threatening voices in clear consciousness; usually lasts less than 6 months
- other – increased depression, increased rate of suicide, sexual problems and pathological jealousy

Example of a psychiatric long case

[This is written in note form, an in an exam.]

HISTORY

Date: 13 May 1995

Personal details:

Name: Simon Long   Marital status: Single
Age: 32   Occupation: Factory worker

Out/inpatient: Inpatient   Section/informal: Section 2

Presenting complaints

A 4-week history of:

1. hearing voices
2. paranoid and grandiose delusions
3. agitation and insomnia

History of presenting complaints

Well until 4 weeks ago. Started with not being able to sleep; noted by brother to be restless, overfamiliar with his neighbours and making inappropriate remarks to them; increased smoking from 10 to 30 cigarettes a day.

Last week, took his workmates out for expensive meals, bought a golden ring for his brother. Transpired he had a loan of £2,000 from bank last week.

Claimed that he had 'made it' to be a multimillionaire and that he would save his workmates and his family from 'needing to earn their bread and butter' in the future.

Says he was told so by 'the One who knows all', and that this was even mentioned in the news recently.

Taken by brother to see GP, who failed to persuade him to see psychiatrist. He was given a prescription of haloperidol 10 mg bd, which he tore up as soon as he left the consulting room.

On day before admission, was sent home by his employer. On that evening, he shouted at a passer-by and tried to run out of the house with a knife, claiming that she was trying to take away his wealth. He was restrained by his brothers, who arrange with his GP for compulsory admission for assessment to take place.

Since admission 3 days ago, has been treated with haloperidol 10 mg tds and procyclidine 5 mg tds.

Past medical history

Nil significant.

Past psychiatric history

September 1993 – admitted informally with severe depression with no apparent cause. Given course of ECT, rapid recovery. Took fluoxetine for 6 months, then stopped. Follow-up by psychiatrists until July 1994.

Medication

Nil.

Allergies

Nil.

Family history

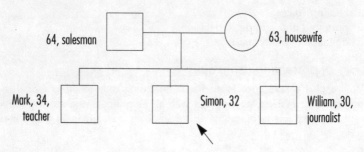

No family history of psychiatric illness.

Social history

Smoking: Usually 10 a day, has increased to 30 a day in last 4 weeks.
Alcohol: At weekends only, less than 3 pints a week.
Illicit drugs: Nil.
General: Factory worker, lives in a three-bedroomed flat with his two brothers. No financial worries.

Personal history

Birth history

Born Norwich, FTND, no perinatal problems.

Developmental history

Normal developmental milestones, no childhood neurotic traits.

Childhood

Described a happy childhood overall. Described both parents as very kind and caring, got on well with brothers except recalls being jealous of his older brother who did better than him academically.

Schooling and further education

Attended Dowell Primary and Secondary School. got on well with teachers and fellow students. Left school aged 16 attaining 4 'O' levels, in maths, English, geography and biology.

Attended a vocational course in car mechanics at Handon Vocational College. Left after 9 months after completing the course.

Occupational history
Cashier at Rapidcash supermarket aged 17–27.
Factory worker at Prosperus Company aged 27 to present. Gets on well with employer and fellow workers.

Psychosexual history
Several girlfriends from age 17 to 25, each lasting a months to a year.
6-year relationship with Amanda from 1988 (aged 25), which ended in December 1993 after his episode of depression. Never engaged or married, no children. Denied that there was any problem in the relationship before his depression.
Has a girlfriend, Sophie (aged 30), for the last 5 months. Sees her frequently and is planning to live together with her.

Forensic history
Nil.

PHYSICAL EXAMINATION

Fit gentleman with no evidence of thyroid disease. No tremor, rigidity or akathisia from present medication. BP 110/70. Rest of examination grossly normal.

MENTAL STATE EXAMINATION

Appearance and behaviour

Dressed in smart bright red clothes. Restless, pacing up and down the room during interview. Talks incessantly. Easily distractible.

Initially friendly; overfamiliar, e.g. patted me on the back several times, saying 'You will do well in this exam, don't worry, boy', but became irritable when interrupted.

Speech

There is much pressure of speech and flights of ideas, with occasional use of clang association, e.g. 'Are you taking your finals? Finals, Arsenal, signals. Yes, they have given me all the signals that I will rule this place soon', 'Do not worry about the examiners, I will give seminars on how to make millions all over the world'.

Mood and affect

Subjectively elated. Objectively elevated mood, but irritable.
Reduced sleep for 4 weeks, appetite and weight normal.

Thought

- *Grandiose thought* – that he will be a millionaire. Thinks it is because he was born destined to be an important person as he has been told so.
- *Paranoid thought* – that there are some unknown people who are trying to deprive him of his 'millions' as they are jealous of him. Unsure of how they are doing that. Had thought of finding out who they are a few days ago, but now 'could not care less, as they will not succeed'.
- Ideas of reference – thinks that the TV news has referred to him several times, when they were talking about 'a millionaire will be born because of this coming weekend's National Lottery'. Thinks that TV only uses the National Lottery as an excuse for referring to him.

Denies thought withdrawal, insertion, broadcasting or passivity feelings.

Perception

Heard both a male and female voice telling him in the 2nd person, 'You will be a millionaire'. Does not know who they are, probably from 'some angels above'.

Congnition

Oriented in time, place and person. Becomes irritable on further assessment.

Insight

Thinks that he is in hospital as his brothers are jealous of him. Denies any illness or need for medication.

SUMMARY

A 32-year-old factory worker with one previous episode of severe depression now presenting with a 4-week history of psychomotor excitation, flights of ideas and paranoid and grandiose delusions. He has no family history of psychiatric illness, and there was no apparent precipitant.

DIFFERENTIAL DIAGNOSIS

The diagnosis for this episode would certainly be mania with psychotic symptoms. Taking into account his previous episode of depression, he appears to suffer from a bipolar affective disorder.

In an exam situation, you may not be able to write or present a case in such detail. In the example above, you can curtail the family and personal history.

8
General Practice

At present, there is no clinical examination in general practice in the finals exam. However, a short chapter is included here for three reasons: the objectives of general practice attachments are different from those of hospital attachments; the style and approach of history taking, physical examination and presentation are different in general practice; and the General Medical Council has, in their report 'Tomorrow's Doctors – Recommendation on Undergraduate Medical Education' (December 1993), recommended extension of the experience of the primary care experience and emphasis of the theme of public health medicine, which will no doubt make general practice feature more prominently both in the undergraduate medical curriculum and its assessments in the future.

Some students appear to think that there is nothing to be gained from their time in general practice, often owing to misconceptions about the objectives of the attachments. They often comment that they 'saw nothing interesting'. The reason for this perception is that they have developed the attitude from their hospital attachments that 'real medicine' involves serious illnesses and heroic treatment. As a result, they get disillusioned and fail to acquire the skills and attitudes that general practice has to offer. Another reason is that some see general practice as 'an aggregate of all hospital specialities, but at an inferior standard'. Again, this is far from the truth.

What general practice can offer to students

- *The process of consultation* – the subject of doctor–patient relationships and the process of consultation have been studied and put into practice probably more by GPs than by any other hospital specialities. Students can learn by observation and discussion with their host GPs.
- *Appreciating illness in the social context and the importance of continuity of care* – general practice is the ideal setting for appreciation of both these issues.
- *Clinical judgement and common sense* – GPs often need to exercise

their clinical judgement without resort to sophisticated diagnostic equipment and investigations. They learn to tolerate uncertainty and to distinguish between the serious and the trivial cases, often without knowing the exact diagnosis.

- *Emergency treatment with minimal support* – students who are 'on call' with GPs may learn how to give first-line emergency treatment (e.g. for hypoglycaemia, acute myocardial infarct or acute asthma), with no support from other staff, minimal equipment and in conditions that may be far from ideal.
- *Health promotion and disease prevention* – students can see primary and secondary prevention in action and critically assess their effects.
- *Working in teams* – although this also occurs in many hospital specialities, it is often much easier for the student to appreciate its advantages and disadvantages in a general practice setting.
- *Management skills* – it is likely that students will learn about financial, resource and staff management, and appreciate the difficulties involved in their observation, from GPs than from hospital consultants.

History taking, examination and presentation

GENERAL ADVICE

You may be asked to see some patients and discuss them with the GPs afterwards. The style of history taking, examination and presentation is quite different from that of hospital specialities.

- *Time available* – the average consultation in a GP surgery lasts between 5 and 10 minutes (although you will be given at least 15–20 minutes!). Hence, the usual 'comprehensive' style of other specialities is inappropriate.
- *Consultation technique* – details of the physical setting of the tables and chairs for doctors and patients (e.g. the patient may sit beside the desk at 45 degrees rather than in a confrontational style facing the doctor) are important in establishing a rapport.

Sensitivity to the 'hidden agenda' is important. Patients' verbal statements of their presenting problems may not be the real or main reasons for the consultation. Recurrent visits for 'trivial symptoms' such as colds may indicate underlying social or marital problems or depression. Patient's worries and fears (e.g. of cancer) may only be hinted at. Observing and interpreting non-verbal communications is important.

HISTORY TAKING, EXAMINATION AND INVESTIGATION

You have the disadvantage compared with the GP that you do not know the patient beforehand and so need to read through the GP's (probably illegible) short notes.

You should concentrate only on the presenting symptoms (and any hidden agenda) and ask about any *relevant* important symptoms and past history, and any points that you think are important for primary or secondary prevention. You should not go through the huge list of headings as in hospital specialities. Similarly, in physical examination, you must know what you are looking for and examine only the systems that are relevant.

Perform investigations only if it necessary and alters your management. Do *not* order 'routine investigations', as some hospital specialists do.

Examples

A previously healthy 35-year-old man complaining of a 3-day history of cough

Ask about frequency and timing (whether night time is more severe) of cough; any sputum, its amount and colour; associated symptoms of fever, shortness of breath and wheezing. Smoking habits should be asked (for health education and illness prevention purposes).

Examine the chest. Take the temperature or perform a peak flow only if you think it is necessary.

Depending on your findings, you probably need not perform any investigations. Your presentation should be short and straightforward.

Mr Y is a 35-year-old labourer with a 3-day history of mild productive cough of yellow sputum. He had no fever, shortness of breath or wheeziness. He smokes 50 cigarettes a day. The chest is clear apart from very occasional crepitation in the left base. I recommend that he joins our 'Stop smoking' group, and I suggest a 5-day course of amoxycillin, and to return if there is no improvement or if deterioration occurs in the meantime.

The GP may want to discuss with you the role of antibiotics, the choice of antibiotics and the best strategies of helping patients to give up smoking.

A 28-year-old on Microgynon (combined oral contraceptive) for past 4 years, who is requesting a repeat prescription

1. history:
   – enquire any problems with its use, presence of withdrawal bleeding, mid-cycle spotting

- check that no contraindications have recently arisen (e.g. history of deep vein thrombosis, severe headache or liver disease)
- enquire about smoking habit (mainly for health promotion purposes – you would still prescribe the pill even if she is smoking)
- enquire the last date of breast examination and cervical smear

2. examination:
   - weight and height
   - blood pressure
   - (breast examination if not done in past 2–3 years)

3. presentation:

   Mrs C is a 28-year-old shopkeeper who has been on Microgynon for the past 4 years and has had no problems with it. There are no contraindications to its use, although she smokes 30 cigarettes a day. She is 3 months overdue for her cervical smear. Her body mass index is 23 (healthy), and her blood pressure is 120/70. I suggest giving her a repeat prescription of Microgynon and booking an appointment in the cervical smear clinic (or performing one now).

A 45-year-old woman presenting with a 5-month history of feeling tired
This case may take longer time than the previous two cases, and the presentation is longer.)

1. history:
   - severity of tiredness, how it started, any associated symptoms
   - recent history of sore throats, colds, sinus problems, contact with others with viral illnesses
   - blood loss (e.g. heavy periods)
   - symptoms of hypothyroidism
   - joint pain, muscle-ache symptoms of connective tissue disease
   - quality and amount of sleep, appetite, weight change and general mood
   - relevant past history
   - social situations at home and work, marital relationship, relationship with children, financial problems
   - use of alcohol and other drugs

2. examination:
   - look for anaemia (conjunctivae)
   - take pulse and blood pressure
   - feel for thyroid gland, look for signs of hypothyroidism
   - look for enlarged lymph nodes (cervical and axillary)
   - feel for abdomen for liver/spleen if necessary

3. investigations:
   - full blood count – for anaemia

– U&E – for renal problems
– ESR
– thyroid function test
– liver function tests, including gamma-GT

4. presentation, for example:

> Mrs R is a 45-year-old housewife who has a 5-month history of tiredness and occasional headache. There are no other associated physical symptoms. She has been feeling low in mood especially in the morning, with loss of appetite, early morning wakening and loss of enjoyment of her usual interest in playing the oboe. She has no ideas of self-harm. Symptoms appear to have started when her son left home for university, and her daughter got married and moved to Aberdeen 6 months ago. She is living with her husband, who is a busy solicitor usually working until 9 pm every day. Over the past few months, her alcohol intake has increased from about 14 units a week to about 30 units a week. Physical examination reveals no abnormality. I suggest we should take blood for FBC, U&E, gamma-GT and thyroid function testing and prescribe a course of the antidepressant fluoxetine. If there is no improvement, we may want to make an appointment for her with our counsellors for cognitive therapy.

The GP may want to take issue with you about the need for these investigations, or about the choice of fluoxetine rather than tricyclic antidepressants.

Future assessment of undergraduates in general practice

Given the General Medical Council's recommendation that 'systems of assessment should be adapted to the new style curriculum ...', it is more than likely that assessments in general practice will play a more important role than at present. How this will be done is not clear. In postgraduate training in general practice, MCQs, modified essay questions, critical reading paper and vivas are used in MRCGP examination, and consideration is being given to videos of consultations and consultation using trained actors as patients. Written audit is used for summary assessments in some vocational training schemes, No doubt, undergraduate assessments may adapt and simplify some of these methods for use in the future.

Index

Abdomen 31
  acute 69–71
  distension 33–4
  examination 37–42
    example 56, 76
  genitourinary system 35–7
  gynaecology 131–2, 145
  intestinal obstruction 68–9
  obstetrics 115, 128
  paediatrics 82, 110
    cystic fibrosis 92
    examination 94–5
    general features 95
    short cases 93–4
  pain 32–3
Abnormal uterine bleeding 135–7
Abortion 133–5
Acute appendicitis 32, 69
Acute pancreatitis 70–1
Affect, psychiatric patients 152, 169
Agnosias 46
Alcohol 15, 149, 164–6
Alimentary system 31–5
Alzheimer's disease 164
Amenorrhoea 136, 137
Anaemia in pregnancy 119–20
Anaesthetic history 59
Anatomical sieve 61
Angina 18
Antenatal care 113
Antenatal investigations, routine 118–19
Antepartum haemorrhage 121–2
Anxiety disorders 161–2
Aortic regurgitation 23
Aortic stenosis 23
Apex beat 23
Appearance, psychiatric patients 151, 169

Appendicitis, acute 32, 69
Apraxias 46
AP shunts 97
Arthritis, rheumatoid 53
Ascites 34
Asthma 92–3
Attention 46, 152
Auscultation
  abdomen 41–2, 95, 116
  cardiovascular system 21–2, 23, 88
  peripheral vascular and venous system 64
  respiratory system 30, 90
  thyroid gland 62
Autoimmune thyroid disease 63

Behaviour, psychiatric patients 151, 169
Birth history 80, 108, 149–50, 168
Blood pressure 21, 23, 88, 120
Bowel habit, change in 34
Bowel infarction 71
Breast 72–4, 132
Breathlessness 19, 25–6
Breath sounds, reduced or absent 30
Bronchial breathing 30

Caesarean section, indications for 125
CAGE questionnaires 15, 165
Calculation, higher cortical function 46
Cancers, gynaecological 140
Cardiovascular system
  diabetes 24
  gynaecology 131, 145
  history 18–21
  obstetrics 115, 127

Cardiovascular system *cont.*
   paediatrics 82, 85–9, 91, 93, 110
   peripheral vascular and venous
      system 63
   physical examination 21–5, 28–9,
      56, 76
Catatonic schizophrenia 158–9
Central nervous system
   obstetrics 116, 128
   paediatrics 82–3, 110
   see also Neurological system
Cerebral palsy 98
Cervical cancer 140
Cervical smear 130, 132
Chest 18, 21–2, 27, 29–30
   paediatrics 86–8, 90–1
Childhood history, psychiatric
      patients 150, 168
Clinical attachments 3, 5–6
Clinical course, preparation for finals
      exam 2–3
Clinical examination, preparation for
      2, 6–10
Clinical judgement, general practice
      171–2
Clubbing 28, 90
Cognition, psychiatric patients
      152–3, 170
Concentration 46, 152
Consultation process, general
      practice 171, 172
Continuity of care 171
Continuous assessment 5–6
Contraception 141–2
Cough 26
Cover test 105
Cranial nerves 50, 57
Crepitation 30
Cyanosis 86, 89
Cystic fibrosis 91–2

Deep vein thrombosis 64–5
Delirium 155–6
Dementia 162–4
Depression 160
Developmental assessment 83, 85,
      99–104, 110
   neurological system 95–6, 97

Developmental history 81, 109,
      150, 168
Diabetes 24–5, 123
Differential diagnosis
   general surgery 77
   groin, lump in 66
   gynaecology 145
   long cases 9–10, 17, 57
   psychiatry 147, 154–5, 170
   short cases 10
Digital pelvic examination 132–3
Distraction test 103–4
Down's syndrome 86, 106
Drug history
   general medicine 14
   general surgery 59, 72, 75
   gynaecology 145
   obstetrics 114, 127
   paediatrics 81, 109
   psychiatry 149, 167
   respiratory history 27
Dysmenorrhoea 137
Dyspepsia 33
Dysphagia 32
Dyspnoea *see* Breathlessness
Dysuria 36

Ectopic pregnancy 70, 133
Education, psychiatric patients 150,
      168
Emergency treatment, general
      practice 172
Equipment 7, 79–80, 84–5, 112
Essay questions, finals exam 1–2, 4
Estimated date of delivery (EDD)
      113
Examiners, interview with 9–10
Eyes 24, 46–7

Family history
   alimentary system 35
   breast 72
   cardiovascular system 20
   general medicine 14–15, 55
   general surgery 59, 75
   genitourinary system 37
   gynaecology 131, 145
   obstetrics 114
   paediatrics 81, 89, 91, 93, 109

Family history *cont.*
  psychiatry 149, 168
  respiratory system 27, 89, 91, 93
  thyroid gland 62
Feedback during clinical course 2
Fetal well-being before labour,
    monitoring of 124
Final clinical exam 7
Finals, hints for preparation 1–5
Forceps delivery, indications for 124
Forensic history, psychiatric patients
    150, 169

Gait, neurological systems 48
Gall bladder 40
Gallstones 70
Gastrointestinal bleeding 38
General anxiety disorder 161–2
General knowledge, higher cortical
    function 45
General Medical Council 171, 175
General medicine 31
  abdomen 31–42
  cardiovascular system 18–24
  diabetes 24–5
  example 54–7
  general advice 11–17
  joints, diseases of 51–3
  neurological system 42–50
  respiratory system 25–31
  skin lesions in systemic disease 54
General practice 171
  future assessments 175
  history taking, examination and
    presentation 172–5
  opportunities for students 171–2
General surgery 58–77
Genitalia, examination 42, 71–2
Genital (uterine) prolapse 143
Genitourinary system 35–7
Gestation 113
Groin, lump in 66, 67
Growth assessment 81–2, 85, 109
Gynaecology 129–46

Haemataemesis 33
Haematuria 36
Haemoptysis 26
Haemorrhage, antepartum 121–2

Hallucinations 152
Health of the Nation 15
Health promotion, general practice
    172
Heart failure 88
Heart valve murmur 22–3, 88
Hebephrenic schizophrenia 158–9
Hepatomegaly 95
Hepatosplenomegaly 95
Hereditary diseases 15, 81
Hernia, suspected 66, 67
Hidden agenda 172
Higher cortical function 45–6
History
  alimentary system 31–5
  breast 72
  cardiovascular system 18–21
  clinical exams, hints for
    preparation 6, 8
  general medicine 11–16, 54–6
  general practice 173–4
  general surgery 58–9, 74–6
  genitourinary system 35–7
  groin, lump in 66
  gynaecology 129–31, 133, 139,
    143–5
  intestinal obstruction 68
  joints, diseases of 51
  neurological system 43–4
  obstetrics 113–14, 119, 121,
    126–7
  paediatrics 78, 79, 80–1
    cardiovascular system 85
    developmental assessment 101
    example 107–9
    neurological system 95–7
    respiratory system 89, 91, 92–3
  peripheral vascular system 63
  psychiatry 147, 148–50, 162–3,
    166–9
  respiratory system 25–8
  thyroid gland 62
Hypertension 120–1
Hypomania 160

Illicit drugs, psychiatry 149
Immunization history, paediatrics
    80, 89, 108
Incontinence 37

Infertility 139–40
Insight, psychiatric patients 153, 170
Inspection
   abdomen 39, 94, 115
   breast 72–3
   chest 21, 29, 86, 90
   groin, lump in 66
   joints 52
   limbs 47, 64
   scrotum 71
   thyroid gland 62
Interests 16
Interviews
   with examiners 9–10
   with patients 7, 8–9
Intestinal obstruction 66–9
Involuntary movements 45

Jaundice 34
Joints, diseases of 51–3
JVP 21, 23

Kidneys 25, 41, 95

Labour 123–5
Language, higher cortical function 46
Last menstrual period (LMP) 113
Lectures 2
Limbs 47–8, 57, 64
Liver 38, 40
Long cases
   clinical exam, preparation for 8–10
   finals exam, preparation for 5
   general medicine 11–17, 54–7
   general surgery 58–60, 74–7
   gynaecology 129–33, 144–6
   obstetrics 112–17, 126–8
   paediatrics 78–84, 107–11
   psychiatry 147–55, 166–70
Lower motor neurone lesions 48

Management skills, general practice 172
Mania 160
Medical history see Past medical history

Medication see Drug history
Memory 45, 152–3
Menstruation history 130, 144
Mental state examination 151–3, 163, 169–70
Mesenteric adenitis 69–70
Mitral regurgitation 23
Mitral stenosis 23
Mock exams 5
Mood, psychiatric patients 151–2, 169
Multiple choice questions (MCQs) 1–2, 4
Myocardial infarction 18

Neurofibromatosis 107
Neurological system 42–3
   cranial nerves, assessment of 50
   diabetes 25
   examination 44–9, 57
   history 43–4
   paediatrics 85, 95–9
   short cases, presentation of 49
   see also Central nervous system
Neurotic disorders 161–2
Notes 2–4

Observation, paediatrics 79, 82–3, 96, 97, 101
Obsessive–compulsive disorder 162
Obstetrics 112–28
Occupation 15
Occupational history, psychiatric patients 150, 169
Oedema 19, 20, 21
Ophthalmoscope, use of own 7
Organic causes of psychiatric disorders 155–6
Orientation 45, 152
Osteoarthritis 53
Ovarian cancer 140

Paediatrics
   abdomen 93–5
   cardiovascular system 85–9
   common syndromes seen in exams 106–7
   developmental assessment 99–104
   equipment list 84–5

Paediatrics *cont.*
  long cases 78–84, 107–11
  neurology 96–9
  respiratory system 89–93
  squints 104–5
Pain relief in labour 124
Palpation
  abdomen 39–41, 94–5, 115–16
  breast 73
  cardiovascular system 21, 23, 86–8
  groin, lump in 66
  joints 52
  limbs 47, 63
  respiratory system 29
  scrotum 71
  thyroid gland 62
Palpitation 19
Pancreatitis, acute 70–1
Panic disorder 162
Paranoid schizophrenia 158–9
Parents of paediatric patients 78,
    101
Pass rates, finals exam 1
Past anaesthetic history 59
Past gynaecological history 114,
    127, 130–1, 144–5
Past medical history
  alimentary system 34–5
  breast 72
  cardiovascular system 20
  general medicine 3, 13, 55
  general surgery 59, 74–5
  genitourinary system 37
  gynaecology 130, 145
  obstetrics 114, 127
  paediatrics 80, 89, 91, 92–3,
    108–9
  peripheral vascular system 63
  psychiatry 148, 167
  respiratory system 27, 89, 91,
    92–3
  thyroid gland 62
Past obstetric history 114, 126,
    130–1, 144
Past psychiatric history 148–9, 167
Past surgical history 59, 74–5
Pathological sieve 61
Pathology 1
Peak flow 30, 90

Pedigree charts 14
Pelvic examination 132–3, 143, 145
Penis 71
Peptic ulcer, perforated 70
Perception, psychiatric patients 152,
    170
Percussion 29–30, 41, 65, 90, 95
Perforated peptic ulcer 70
Performance peak flow 30
Pericarditis 18
Perinatal mortality, factors
    increasing risk of 125
Peripheral vascular and venous
    system 63–5
Peritonitis 69
Personal details
  general medicine 11, 54
  general surgery 58, 74
  gynaecology 129, 144
  obstetrics 113, 126
  paediatrics 80, 107
  psychiatry 148, 166–7
Personal history, psychiatric patients
    149–50, 168–9
Pharmacology 2
Phobic anxiety disorder 161
Physical examination
  abdomen 37–42
  breast 72–3
  cardiovascular system 21–4
  clinical exams, hints for 6, 8, 9
  general medicine 16–17, 56–7
  general practice 173, 174
  general surgery 59, 76
  gynaecology 131–3, 143, 145–6
  intestinal obstruction 68–9
  joints, diseases of 52
  male genitalia 71–2
  neurological system 44–9
  obstetrics 115–16, 119, 127–8
  paediatrics 78–9, 81–3, 109–10
    abdomen 94–5
    asthma 93
    cystic fibrosis 91–2
    developmental assessment
      101–2
    neurological system 97–8
  peripheral vascular and venous
    system 63–5

Physical examination *cont.*
  psychiatry 150–1, 169
  respiratory system 28–30
  thyroid gland 62
Pleural rub 30
Polyhydramnios 115
Polyuria 36
Postgraduate exams, finals as
    practice for 1
Postoperative cases 60
Power, limbs 48
Practicals, hints for 1
Pre-eclampsia 120–1
Premorbid personality 150
Preoperative cases 60
Preparation, hints for 1–10, 153
Presentation of cases
  abdomen 42
  cardiovascular system 24
  clinical exams 7, 8–9
  continuous assessment 6
  general medicine 17
  general practice 173, 174, 175
  general surgery 60
  gynaecology 133, 145
  neurological system 49
  obstetrics 116–17
  paediatrics 79, 83–4, 88–91,
    98–9, 102–3
  peripheral vascular and venous
    system 64
  psychiatry 153–5, 170
  respiratory system 31
Presenting complaint(s)
  alimentary system 31–4
  cardiovascular system 18–20
  general medicine 11–12, 54–5
  general surgery 58–9, 74
  genitourinary system 35–7
  groin, lump in 66
  gynaecology 129–30, 143, 144
  paediatrics 80, 89, 91, 92, 108
  peripheral vascular system 63, 64
  psychiatry 148, 167
  respiratory system 25–7
  thyroid gland 62
Preventive medicine 15, 172
Pseudo-squints 105
Psychiatry 147–70

Psychosexual history, psychiatric
    patients, 150, 169
Pulmonary oedema 19
Pulmonary stenosis 23
Pulse 21, 23, 86
Pupillary abnormalities 46
Pylonephritis 70

Rapport with patients 78, 172
Rectal bleeding 34
Rectal examination 42, 59
Reflex, limbs 48
Remote memory 45
Renal colic 70
Resits 5
Respiratory system
  gynaecology 131, 145
  history 25–8
  obstetrics 115, 128
  paediatrics 82, 85, 89–93, 110
  peripheral vascular and venous
    system 63
  physical examination 28–30, 56,
    76
  presentation of short cases 31
Revision 3–7
Rhesus incompatibility 120
Rheumatoid arthritis 53
Romberg's sign 49
Routine antenatal investigations
    118–19
Ruptured ectopic pregnancy 70

Salpingitis 70
Schizophrenia 156–7, 158–9
Schooling, psychiatric patients 150,
    168
Scrotum 71–2
Seminars 2
Sexual history 131
Short answers, finals exam 1–2, 4
Short cases
  clinical exam, hints for 10
  finals exam, hints for 5
  general surgery 60–74
  neurological system 49
  paediatrics 86–91, 93–4, 104
  psychiatry 147
  respiratory system 31

Sigmoid diverticulitis 70
Skin 24, 54
Sleep, importance of 7
Smoking history 15
Social context of illness 171
Social history
   alimentary system 35
   cardiovascular system 20
   general medicine 15–16, 56
   general surgery 59, 75–6
   genitourinary system 37
   gynaecology 131, 143, 145
   obstetrics 114, 127
   paediatrics 81, 89, 93, 109
   peripheral vascular system 63
   psychiatry 149, 168
   respiratory system 28, 89, 93
Social life, balanced 2, 4–5
Speculum examination 132
Speech, psychiatric patients 151,
   169
Spleen 41
Sputum 26
Squints 85, 104–5
Stethoscope, use of own 7
Stool characteristics and causes 34
Stridor 27
Study groups 4
Suicide, assessing risk of 157, 161
Summary of case 8–9
   general medicine 17, 57
   general surgery 60, 76
   gynaecology 133, 145
   obstetrics 116–17, 128
   paediatrics 83–4, 110–11
   psychiatry 153–4, 170
Surge–Weber syndrome 107
Surgical history 59, 74–5
Swelling, short case examination
   60–1
Systemic enquiries 16, 76

Teamwork, general practice 172
Tenderness, abdominal 40
Termination 133–5

Textbooks 2–6
Therapeutic abortion 134–5
Therapeutics 2
Thought, psychiatric patients 152,
   170
Thyroid gland 62–3
Time factors
   clinical exams 7, 8, 10
   general practice 172
   general surgery 58
   gynaecology 129
   history taking 13, 16
   obstetrics 112
   psychiatry 147
Trendleburg test 65
Tricuspid regurgitation 23
Tricuspid stenosis 23
Tuberous sclerosis 107
Turner's syndrome 86, 106

Unemployment 15
Upper motor neurone lesions 48
Urinary symptoms 35
Urinary tract disorder 38
Urine testing 17, 42
   obstetrics 116, 118, 128
   paediatrics 83
Uterine bleeding, abnormal 135–7
Uterine cancer 140
Uterine prolapse 143

Vaginal discharge 138
Vaginal examination 116, 128
Varicose veins 65
Vascular dementia 164
Vascular and venous system,
   peripheral 63–5
Visual field abnormalities 46–7
Viva, hints for 1–2
Vomiting 33

Ward rounds 6
Week before finals 4–5
Wheeze 27, 30

Anabella
DARK SU

CW00487004

Dark Su
(An Indecency Suites Novella #2)

Randers
And
Trant

Copyright: Anabella Roscoff 2019

Anabella Roscoff
DARK SURRENDER

This is a work of fiction. Names, characters, places, brands, media and incidents are either the product of the author's imagination or are used fictitiously. The author acknowledges the trademarked status and trademark owners of various products, bands, and/or restaurants referenced in this work of fiction, which have been used without permission. The publication/use of those trademarks is not authorized, associated with, or sponsored by the trademark owners.

License Notes

The Indecency

Suites

Anabella Roscoff
DARK SURRENDER

~ Book 2 ~

Chapter 1

Lilly

My fingers flick off the lights in the hall, hands pulling the door closed behind me. He'll be there soon with any luck. I got a text a while back from him to tell me the plane had been delayed and that he was on route, he'd be about an hour late. I was just leaving for the cabin when it came in, so I sat and waited here a bit longer. I can't wait anymore. Why should I? I thought staying here would give me less time alone out in those woods, but I'm so hungry for him, and I've denied myself long enough.

I've tried giving it all up, but just a
few times a year I need someone who knows
exactly what he's doing. And they're non-
toxic. Clean. Which is more than can be said
for some of the locals round here. It's not like
I'm a complete hussy. They're thorough, too.
Health checks and paperwork show they're
regularly passed as safe to do their work. This
small town full of married men and ineligible
bachelors I'm in is draining on a woman's
libido. Okay, so I get a reprieve every now
and then when I travel to the city, and I make
the very most of that, but living with my mom
and dad at the age of twenty six is not helping
me out in the man zone.

I walk to the car, crossing over the
ridiculous stepping stones mom had put in last
week. At least I've got money to get a place
with at some point. The job pays damn well,
even if it has brought me back to this town I
grew up in, but I did not go through medical

school to live at home with my parents. Thank god they've gone out for the night, because that's given me chance to just leave a note saying I'm staying with a friend. The interrogation would have been horrendous if they'd been here.

Another thing to not love about being at home again.

I check my watch and open the car door, ready to make my way over to the lakeside cabin I've booked for the weekend. Heath Randers is meeting me there. That's his name. Not that I'll get him all weekend, but the thought would be nice if it was ever achievable. It's not, unfortunately. And I so wish it was. Perhaps then I could lose this professional attitude I've come to apply to myself permanently. Enjoy life and relax in the rather lewd thoughts I have most of the day.

The engine starts and I'm out on the road as quick as I can, speeding the corners to get there. It's not far away, but something about doing the things Heath gets me to do in my mom and dad's house just seems repulsive. He's something out of this world, and the only one I've used so far. The service offers all kinds, but his profile stood out last year when I saw him. Tall, broad, muscular. Something about his eyes, as well. They seemed nasty behind a preppy outlook. And he is nasty. *Very.* It starts out sweet enough, pleasant words from an educated man, but then he starts getting his bag of toys out, and what those toys can do? My god. I almost fainted last time. That was the first time.

This is the second time.

The sky is black as coal as I keep driving through the country side, roads winding deeper into the woods. I squint a little, trying to get a good view without streetlamps to help me, and slow as the ground becomes bumpy underneath the tyres. It's eerie out here. Nothing but the dim light of the moon to light my way deeper into these trees. Thankfully, the lake comes into view after a few minutes, the expanse of it riding out to the east into yet more darkness. I crawl the edge of it, finally beginning to see some glimmer of light in the distance, and smile.

Thank god I've made it alive without launching myself into the inky waters.

The wheels pull to a stop as arrive and park, and I sweep the outside area looking for where his car might be. It still isn't here that I can see. No matter, he'll turn up soon enough. The service prides itself on never letting anyone down. I was told about it by a colleague in med school. A rich colleague. She said it was the best thing she'd ever spent money on. And then told me that a man called Bolton Bradley was exceptionally good. I looked him over first, but, like I said, Heath stood out from all the rest, including the other thirty I perused that night.

I get out and head up the rickety old path, carrying my overnight bag with me, and dig in my pockets for the keys to get in. A crack sounds out somewhere, enough to have me spinning on myself before I reach the porch. There's nothing that I can see. Nothing but that eerie stillness and the sound of water gently lapping the shore.

"Heath?" I call out, quietly, nerves rattling me.

No more noise comes, though, so I turn and head for the cabin again.

Chapter 2

Heath

I'd forgotten what she was like, self-assured little madam that she is. She's attractive. Long hair, mostly tied up in a bun or chignon. Tonight she's in jeans and boots, as if I didn't even warrant correct dress etiquette. I dodge the trees to the right and watch as she hovers on the path, unsure what's around her. I'm around her, and my part here for the night is to give madam a lesson in manners. The first part of which will be removing those disgusting things she's chosen to wear for our date.

That's what this is to me.

A date.

I accept or decline an invitation with no thought to the money involved. I don't need it. Never have done. And because of my last time with her I chose to accept. She was good, amenable to my fondling and arousal. Got my cock off four times. Unusual for me in two hours. Perhaps it was the way she sucked it, maybe even the things she let me put inside her. Which were despicable and many.

And horny as fuck.

I crack another branch underfoot purposely, and watch as she scuttles around the path she's on leading up to the cabin. It's a hike for her up to it, and so I silently creep through the undergrowth wondering what screwed up thing I can use to torment her into submission. She doesn't like it much. She's one of the confident types, unwilling, for whatever reason, to bow down and accept her surrender for a few hours. Silly girl. Life is so

much simpler when one accepts one's fate.
And this one's fate is in my hands tonight.

She puts the holdall she's carrying on
the ground at one point and lifts her phone
into the air, searching for signal presumably.
There isn't any here that I'm aware of, and
that's a lovely thing for me. She'll be
disarmed by it, worried that she's not in
control of something. She's not. Not for two
hours. I am.

Another crack underfoot and her head
spins to the sound of me, hands grabbing at
her bag again and feet running up the rocky
path. Amusing. I chuckle to myself and head
round the back of the place, dropping my
balaclava down to mask me and pulling the
thin, leather gloves on. All black now. Black
as this night around us and ready to show her
a new path other than that confidence she
portrays. Confidence has no sense of fear, and
fear is what she needs. A little excitement in

her life to remind her that not everything in this world should be ordered to within an inch of its life.

The door closes as she finds her way in. I hope she feels happy there for a moment or two. Safe. It'll help the rest come so much easier when I get my hands on her skin. I carry on to the back and climb up through the bedroom window, loosing the catch I left half open earlier. I've already been in, picked the locks and had a good look around before she got here just to set this scene up correctly for her entitled little bottom. No plane journeys, no delay like I told her about. I've had this planned since the moment she sent her message through the system 3 months ago. It was rude:

Meet on the 17th June. 8pm.
Lake Taldo Retreat, Maine. Cabin 14.

No asking. No pleasant conversation to persuade me into her bidding. Just those details and a smug sense of satisfaction that I would do as I was told. I replied with nothing more than an agreement, a sneer on my face as I sent it.

Bitch.

The sound of clattering halts me as I get to the main door into the hall, her mutterings about something proving useful to cloud any noise, and then she goes to the stereo system and puts some music on. It's tranquil, presumably soothing to her fearful nerves. My foot kicks the back of the door I'm behind, loud enough that she'll hear it and come investigate. Entitled little bitch will not forget this night, and she'll damn well apologise for her manner when it's finished, too.

DARK SURRENDER

The sound of her footsteps approaching make me smile and stay back, ready to get on with what I'm here for. The moment she's through the door I'm on her, grabbing her arm and spinning her so her back is against my chest. She struggles and squawks, arms and legs trying to beat into me so she can run. She's not running anywhere for a while, and me throwing her onto the bed harshly proves my point. I slam the door, picking out the handcuffs from my pocket, and hurry towards her. She screams loud enough for the goddamn world to hear, hands and legs wheeling like a banshee to get away. But there's no one here to save her now. She's alone, and me dodging to counter every move she makes only seems to be evoking a fear that soothes my own soul.

She's smothered before she gets the next scream out, one hand ratcheted by the cuff to the bed post and the other held tight in my grip. Nice. Effective. I can smell her fear from here, see it in the wide blue eyes that are near hysterical from the attack she's under. She spits at me, body still trying to struggle. Good girl. She's trying, trying to get away from the rapist. Her mother would be proud, I'm sure. But me? I find the spitting a touch rude, and the increased pressure and growl that comes from my throat proves my annoyance. She lays there under me, shutting her pretty little mouth down quick enough now I'm physically hurting her. It wakes my cock up, arousing the sadist in me. I try not to be these days. Not always good for the job, but fuck it with this one. She deserves a good hiding.

"Please," she says, quietly, trying to scuttle again. I cover the move and reach into my pocket for more cuffs, then flip her over onto her front. I'd like to ask her what she's

begging for, but that would give me away.
"Please. Don't. What do you want?" she says.

I barely stop the laugh that wants to come out, because what does she think a rapist wants? Her cunt, is what I want. I want it on my mouth, around my fingers, and eventually having my cock rammed into it as she howls out in terror.

I'm going to get all that, too.

But first I'm going to play.

And she's going to scream some more.

Chapter 3

Lilly

O h god. Why isn't he here yet? I struggle again, trying to counter this man's weight on me, but I can't get out from under him. He's so heavy on me, all over me. I pant, breathless from the fight I tried to put up. It's useless. There's no way I'm going to get out of this. My eyes flick around, looking at the door and trying to listen for a car arriving. Perhaps if Heath can get here quick enough, he'll be able to stop this happening.

Anabella Roscoff
DARK SURRENDER

They always told me to submit if someone tried this, that being aggressive only winds them up more and makes it more pleasurable for them. A gulp of fear tries to calm my limbs down, hoping that holds true. Perhaps it does, but it's not stopping my whole body vibrate with fear, as he moves above me. I can hear his breath, feel his cock digging into my thigh, as he rubs himself into me.

Slowly he pulls my free arm wide, another cuff being clicked into place around my wrist. I'm shunted by his legs, his hand dragging my body up the bed to get my arm to the other bedpost. The metal clicking into place signals my capture, no matter how much I tried to pull back from it happening. Tears wet my eyes, mouth buried in the pillow as I feel him move back off me. There's nothing I can do now.

No way of getting out of whatever he's got planned.

Unless Heath hurries.

"Someone's coming," I spit out, trying to look back and get a glance at him.

All I see is a mask of black and a body encased in the same colour. He just stands there and looks me over, no features to give his identity away. The tears that were just arriving begin to tumble out of me, knowing what's going to happen next. My head turns into the sheets, muffling my mouths want to protest and scream, and hiding my tears. What good will it do? No one's here but me and him. And I will not let him see me panic. I'll remain calm, try to send my head off somewhere else until Heath arrives.

Rustling begins in the background, a zipper being drawn down. My whole body tenses as I imagine his fly coming down, his fingers getting a cock out to rape me with.

DARK SURRENDER

Sickness floods my stomach, warning me to prepare for the worst. And then his hands start tugging at the jeans covering me, pulling them down to below my backside. I retch a little, bile coming up my throat, and then cough it away.

"No, please," mumbles out of me, more tears spilling from my eyes.

He doesn't respond, just keeps tugging until both my jeans and panties are around my knees. I clamp my thighs as tightly as I can, hoping I can keep him out of me somehow. My head shakes, knowing I won't be able to. I've got no hope of managing my way through this, other than pretending it isn't happening. "Heath!" shouts out of me. It's one last attempt at getting helped somehow. No one answers. I'm alone.

I don't know what happens next. I'm tugged and moved around slightly, knees pushed up under me. I try to fight it, try struggling against it, but my head is shoved into the pillow to remind me of his strength. I whimper at it, the tension in my body finally giving up at that last show of control. There's nothing left for me to do but accept and try to ignore. So I do, eyes squeezing tightly and mouth clamping closed. That's all he's getting from me. No screams. No fear to wind him further up. I'll pretend it isn't happening, perhaps imagine it is Heath rather than a stranger.

Something touches my thigh, and I yelp and move, no ability to hide the sense of fear. Oh god, it's … I don't know what it is. It's cold, hard. I shake my head and close my mouth again, refusing to let this beat me. He runs it across my backside, trailing it around the area and dipping it lower with each brush on my skin. My knees move me again the moment it slides over the exposed area between my thighs. *No.* My mind tries to get me away from what's happening, but he pushes slightly, dragging and shoving it towards my insides. Everything in me clamps – thighs, calves, arms braced - everything.

A slickness sounds, as he finally gets whatever it is where he wants it. It increases the bile that wants to race from my stomach. I'm wet, my body excited by the possibility, as he slides it around me. I heave again, unable to accept my reaction to this degenerate behaviour, and the moment I do something is forced inside me. My mouth opens at the impact, eyes widening immediately, as I feel it going deeper. It keeps going, then slowly pulls out. Ridges. I can feel ridges on it, as he drives it back in again all the way to the hilt. I look at the metal bedframe, willing myself to not respond, as I'm shunted towards it, but the quivering in my legs begins as the feeling intensifies. Oh god, I'm enjoying it.

I cough, trying to ignore the sensation, but he repeats the move over and over again, making me moan involuntarily. It's harsh, the movement made with a firm hand, but it's not painful. I expected that. Expected to be held down and have his cock rammed into me quickly, hands clawing at me and foul breath in my face, but this is …

A growl sounds out from him. Low and animalistic. It makes me tense, as he increases the force of the instrument and shoves it harder. I gulp at the feel of it, legs shaking again as he leans over me. I can feel his breath at my back, and his hand jostling my top up, exposing more of my skin. Teeth bite in instantly, making me howl out in pain, but my backside keeps moving to allow him further inside me. My thighs even loosen with the next forge inwards, another moan coming from my mouth. I'm going to cum, and his gloved hand travelling beneath my top to find my nipple severely doesn't stop the sensation finding more strength. I writhe at the feeling, trying to shake it off and make it stay away from the moment.

Something changes in the rhythm he's creating, and I feel myself longing for him to go back to what he *was* doing. The feel of orgasm disperses instantly, bringing me back to the fact that I'm being I'm being taken with force, held fast. Yet he's doing everything I need in the exact way I need it. It's haunting my mind with memories of good sex, consensual sex, and I feel myself needing more of the same thing again. A whimper and mewl seem to leave me at the same time, some annoyance at the impact being taken from me. A hard hand slaps down on my backside the second the sound leaves my lips, shunting me forward. I gasp at it, and then feel lost the moment he draws whatever is inside me out.

I'm left like that – exposed and dripping. I can feel that, too, wetness and my own juices flowing down the inside of my thighs. It makes another whimper come from me, disgust with my own neediness filling me with self-loathing, and I look down at the crumpled pillows to let some of the tears fill my eyes. I'm enjoying this.

Enjoying being taken.

Chapter 4

Heath

She's surprised me with this attitude of hers. I expected far more spitting and swearing to come from her. Seems she likes a little rough. She's certainly showing it with the amount of liquid dribbling down her desperate little thighs. Even now, as I watch and make her wait, she hovers like a needy little thing, her ass waving in my face. My tongue licks over my lips, teeth ready for a little more fun. She smells good, too. Warm. Wet. Sweet hints of her arousal flooding my senses and winding up the old bastard in me.

Only one hit, though. One hit for the sweet little Lilly who's being reminded what a dirty little madam she really is under that insolence of hers. I'd like more but that's not what I'm here for today. She's taking what I give and nothing else.

I can't help myself but try tasting that sweetness of hers. My mouth gets closer to her cunt, ready to draw my tongue over her and taste the flavour I've not had for a while. Perhaps fear will increase the sweet nectar's offering, enthuse it. I lap quietly at first, drawing from her clit through to her ass. She's sodden, all of it pouring out of her asking for my cock. I find the entrance to her and thrust in harder, moving my tongue in small circles to lap everything out of her before I ram my cock home. I want her dry, all the ease of slide removed so she can feel the cock hammering her. She might know then. The moment I start fucking her she'll be reminded of my size, the

way I use this cock she pants for every damn
time.

My hand reaches for the black dildo
again, as I tear little nips at her cunt and pull
the skin taught with my teeth, enjoying the
thought of putting in in her ass as I fuck her. I
can rest my abs on it, make it mimic the
fucking I give her pussy. Maybe she won't
know it's me then. She moans back at me,
cunt beginning to grind in my face. Dirty little
thing. Sweet. I could carry on for hours, but
my cock needs release before I can keep going
again. The drive was long to get here, and her
ass in my face is making me ravenous to
empty my load into her cunt first time round.

I press the dildo onto her skin again,
letting it roll down the crack of her ass
towards her opening. She bucks for it, and me,
and a healthy dose of humiliation comes with
the tone of her whimper. I like that sound. I
make the move happen again, and again, until

her thighs loosen completely and she tries to widen those knees for me. My head moves back, watching as she fidgets and undulates in front of me, nothing to find any purchase on. I give her something with the increase in pressure on the glass dildo, right over a hole she doesn't want me to go in. That's on her profile. No anal stimulation. Fuck that. Madam wants anything I give her now. And she's being raped, what does she expect? I'm going to adhere to rules? That's not going to happen anymore. Not that she knows who's raping her.

She quivers at the feel of pressure on her ass, but doesn't move any further than a slight shuffling of her knees. It intrigues me given her profile statement, making me unzip slowly and pull my rigid cock out. Perhaps madam's got a history that needs investigating, and after this fucking happens maybe I'll give a damn, but at the moment I want an apology and nothing more.

I push harder and move myself so I can ready myself to get up inside her. She moans and groans, ass fidgeting, as I keep putting pressure on it and watch as she begins expanding for me. I wait, a half hover, offering a reprieve if she really wants it, before not giving a fuck and pushing it all the way in. She groans and raises her ass further into the air, face squashed into the pillows and muffling her words. They mutter and mumble, though. A litany of them coming from her in her delirium. I could get all up inside that emotion, lose myself in her charms now I know she's up for rough and destructive. She's always been a looker. Elegant. Intelligent. Perfect and crisp. But this little tiger coming out to play with me?

I could wile weeks away inside that.

"Please," she mutters.

Please. She's begging for me now. The word soothes my soul, bringing with it connotations of obscenity and vulgarity. No one loves a vulgar little whore more than me. I yank the dildo nearly out, bitterly, letting the ridges do the job they're designed for, and then push it back in just as forcefully. Her whole body shudders and rocks, crafting my poetry with the same look. She's a work of art now for me. A blank canvas to turn into stripes of degradation for me to play with.

"Please," she splutters, rising her ass backwards for more depth.

I move closer towards her, pushing it to its very deepest and giving my own cock a couple of draws to line it up. Everything's open for me. I could ram this cock wherever I choose to and she'd still moan and beg for it now. This isn't rape for her anymore. Its energy and orgasms, just the way I prefer my sex. I fuck like that with no care to how much pleasure is received by the recipient, only that they moan to help get me off. And this one moans well, even better this time around.

My cock laps the core of her, sliding through the sluice of liquid that's coming again. Fuck, I wanted her dry. I grab at the sheet, wiping her off and shoving some of it up inside her to parch that area of pleasantries. She's wound up the animal now, the one who brings pain with him and prefers the sound of agony while he's fucking.

The moment I'm satisfied with the effort, I shunt straight at the waiting hole and cover the dildo with my stomach. She tries to buckle under the force of both things, a decadent scream sounding out in the room because of the pain. I don't let her. My hand wraps under her frame to lift her back up to me. Open is what I want. If I have to damn well hold her up to keep her open, I'll do it to get what I want out of this fuck.

Chapter 5

Lilly

I'm so full. I can't breathe. Everything is full to bursting and it's … painful. No, not painful. Throbbing. He's all I can feel. I don't know where I begin and he ends now. I don't even know what that is in my backside, but it burns as he nudges it slightly. He's just waiting in me. Barely any movement at all. I shake my head, trying to find clarity in whatever is happening. I said please. Begged him for more of whatever this is, regardless of the situation I'm in. A choked sob leaves my lips, tears still coming from my eyes gently, as I tug at the handcuffs keeping me locked in place.

It's a lie – the capture. I'm not struggling anymore, haven't done since his tongue started going inside of me. I'm turned on, ready for more of this situation. Even before that I was stimulated, ready to cum if he'd have kept going with that rhythm. He's kept me on the precipice of that, though. Not letting me get any momentum up again.

His cock inches out slowly. I know it's a cock this time. It's softer than the other thing, wider too. It glides and slides rather than the other thing that bumps and batters against me. And that thing is in my backside, buried deep in there. I didn't even protest, too wound up in whatever sick desire this is to object. I wish I could see his face, know the man who's causing this reaction in me and thank him for it.

A gurgled breath puffs out of me as he buries his cock back in me again, shunting the other thing at the same time. I don't even know how to describe the feeling. Full is all I've got. Consumed maybe. I pant, trying to get a sense of rhythm in his attack as it starts to progress. It's on going, the force and weight beginning to pick up in intensity with every drive into me. My cheek rests on the pillows, neck straining to get me up higher. I want my hands un-cuffed so I can lift myself and get a better angle, a deeper one.

His hands roam, as his forearms hold me up a small amount, pinching at my nipples through my bra. They twist and tug as he keeps spearing into me, both objects making me groan and buck in his hold. I'm lost in whatever delusional thing this is, moaning for more with every next breath I can manage to find. More comes at me. More strength. More aggression in every next shunt. I'm collapsed in his hold, unable to move other than what he wants me to do. One gloved hand leaves me and braces itself on the bed in my line of view. I watch it straining and gripping onto the sheets as he keeps hammering away silently. It grips tighter and tighter, screwing up into a fist. It's just like the orgasm that's chasing through me now, tension forcing it quicker and harder as he keeps banging on my backside and driving his cock deeper and deeper. There's nowhere else for it to go that out of my mouth, and those ridges inside me combined with the powerful thrusts that keep coming, send a new wave of frenzy over my skin.

I moan, and the ache becomes unbearable the harder and faster he pushes me. It's like the whole world seems to be evaporating, nothing else but sensation and his hand in my eye-line. Grunts come from him, ones that only enthuse this wanton display of desire in me. I listen to them, letting them spur me on to the end destination with no care to the thought of what's happening. They increase in strength along with his manic fucking, more aggressive growls of pleasure coming from him every time he manages to find new depths to plunder.

Everything tenses in me suddenly, and I feel the relief begin washing over my entire frame from the attack. I stare at the hand and let it come over me, crashing into some kind of hysterical need for more and more of it to channel though me. I want his cum in me, want the feel of that last final drive in to deliver his semen into something that protested then begged. And I want the sound, too. I want a roar of success to leave his throat and tell me I did well under his attack. That I took this and pleased him.

Tears come again at that thought, disgust mixing with the colours that are clouding my vision and swimming through my mind. I'm coming under him, coming undone and enjoying it. Who thinks like that in the middle of this? I do, it seems. And I want him to carry on after this is done. I want him to keep me tied up and force my surrender time and time again until I'm nothing but memories and shaking limbs.

Nothing stops when I feel the last of my orgasm dissipate. My stomach gets dropped until I'm flat on the bed, and he continues to use me in a new position, changing the intensity of the drives in. His hand shoves in between my legs, pushing my knees out to splayed and open so he can run his gloved hand over my tender offering. I sense him rubbing his cock on his own leather gloved hand, the fingers giving me something to put my clitoris against as he keeps fucking into me.

"Again," growls out of his lips at my ear.

I gasp at the sound of his voice, for some reason more scared of that than what's happening. It causes the thought of more orgasms to come, though. Is that what he means? I don't know, but I grind my clitoris on his hand as the weight of the thing in my backside drives in deeper. I'm so repulsed with myself that I close my eyes again and pray that I'll never have to think about it again, certainly not with this sense of desire attached to the memory. Everything slows slightly the moment I do. The shunts in - deeper and less aggressive. The weight - left inside me longer, small movements that are rigid and fast rather than the long exaggerated fucking I've been under. It becomes smooth and fluid, like a wire between us connects the momentum and forces two bodies into doing what they shouldn't be doing. "Make yourself cum, Lilly." My eyes fly open, instantly recognising the voice this time.

Heath.

Chapter 6

Heath

She tries to get her pretty little face turning back to look at me, and I find my hand slapping at it to get it back to the pillow where it belongs. I'm pissed at myself now. I shouldn't have spoken, but the feel of her around my cock and the breathy little groans she kept making got me all fucking verbal. My cock shunts in hard, ready to break her open for being rude to me with that message. She squeals at the ferocity of it, puffing out air as I keep riding in to bring myself on. The sound enthuses me back to my purpose, and I slap at her cheek again, wanting an apology out of her entitled little mouth before I honour her with my cum inside her.

"Apologise," grates out of me.

Not that she'll know what for, but I'm so close to coming now I'm hardly managing to keep this going any longer. I need to get the words from her, make her realise that I will not be ordered by anyone. She shifts and grinds down onto my hand, suddenly wild with her movements now she knows it's me. It forces the cum inside me to take over, forging its way from my balls and into the depths of a place that doesn't deserve it yet.

I pull out and kneel back on the bed, withdrawing all touch from her and yanking the dildo from her ass in the same move. Bitch will not get another orgasm. Not now. Not from me, anyway. Still, she grinds on the bed, though, mewling and purring like the little tiger she's become. My own hand works faster on my cock, grunts coming as I stare at her writhing around, ass in the air and jeans round her ankles. It works harder and faster with each next move of her body, enthused by the shameless state she's in. Hair falling over her face, pink cheeks and a swollen cunt up on offer for me.

My teeth launch at it, hand bracing me on all fours, as I keep pumping cock, and I bite hard into tender flesh. She screams at that and tries to scurry away, amusing me with the sound of fear again. I tear in some more, and then bite in another way until the screams keep coming and the settled sense of safety she felt has left again. Fuck that. She's not safe here. Never was with me on the loose and all riled up.

Rude bitch.

"I'm sorry!" she shouts out.

Good. She should be.

The apology is enough to have me unable to hold back any longer, and I rear up over her back to empty onto that rather than the place she wants me to be. It flows out of me in waves, grunts coming with each next spurt on creamy white skin. She undulates beneath it, arms and body trying to find a way of accepting this nature I'm giving to her. Fuck the money. Fuck the rules I'm supposed to abide by. T can try reprimanding me for it at some point, probably while she's underneath me screaming her voice out, too.

Done.

For now.

Breath heaves into me, as I regain my breathing, and I back up off the bed to get to the floor again. "You're an entitled little bitch, Lilly Trant," grumbles out of me, as I reach for the bag I brought earlier in the evening.

My hand pulls the balaclava off my head, and cool air instantly sends some relief from the heat I've been in. I smile at the contents of the bag and dig into it for rope and other goods to enthuse more apologies. She'll learn well tonight. I've got nowhere else to be for two days, and women who forget their manners should be shown who they're attempting to order around. Including T the next time I get my hands on her vicious little tongue. That bitch can eat up her phone call asking where I am and if I've finished. I answer to no one.

"Heath?"

That's the second time she's said my name now. I like it. I don't know why. I normally detest my name from their lips, but with her, after this fucking, and the sense of nerves in her now, I'm all over enjoying the sound of it a while longer.

"What did you apologize for?" I ask, picking out a short reed cane.

She's looks back at me, a frown on her brow as she glances at the cane I'm holding.

"What?"

"The apology, what for?"

"I don't know," she stutters out. She should. I want her to know, want her to understand who she's hired for the evening. She tugs at the handcuffs, her body trying to roll away from my advance. "I don't know what any of this has been, Heath, but that's not going anywhere near me." Oh yes it is. "And there's no way I'm paying if…"

I chuckle and watch her watch me, my own fingers desperate to touch this new thing I've found to play with. "Did you like the rape-play?"

"No." I stare. Waiting. She fidgets under my scrutiny, no doubt struggling to admit she wanted what she just got. "Yes then, but…" She twists, eyes trained on the cane still. "I mean... that's not what you're booked for and..."

"This wasn't a booking the moment you were rude to me."

"When?"

"When you ordered me to come here. The message? Rude."

Her eyes widen some more, watching as I start pulling my thin black shirt off to expose my skin. Good. I like that, too. It's been a while since I've been ogled like this. Four months I think since the last request I accepted. "Heath, I don't know what you're playing at but this has to stop. Unlatch these cuffs and leave."

"No."

"This is ..." Her body scurries upwards, knees pulling up into herself to try and get away. I smirk at the move and unbuckle my belt, ready to have a lot more fun before the night is through. "This is not right."

"Tell me you didn't like what I just gave you." Her mouth opens, eyes looking, as I draw my cock out again and give it a few tugs. "Tell me you don't want more and I'll walk out." Her eyes stay transfixed on my hand working cock, lips licking over her tongue without her knowing. "Be careful, though, little Lilly. You're not paying for a thing tonight. Or tomorrow if you play your cards right. Make sure you don't blow your chance out the window."

She doesn't say anything else. She just squirms and keeps watching my hand.

Good. I'll take that a yes.

Chapter 7

Lilly

I wish I knew what I was doing, but I seemingly don't. I'm here, chained up to bedposts, with my jeans round my ankles and Heath coming at me holding, what looks like, a headmaster's cane. I gulp, knowing I should be saying no. He told me to say it. Asked me to tell him I didn't want this and then he'd leave. I can't get the words out, though. My mouth has stayed open as I watch him stroke his cock, eyes locked on that and the trail of black hair that led down to it. Everything about him is so dark, swarthy. And

now I know it's him, even though I don't
know this version of him, I'm utterly lost as to
how to say no.

He walks to the edge of the bed and
waits some more, as if giving me a chance to
find the words I'm looking for and decline his
offer. I won't. Even if I knew how to say them
in this moment, I can't deny the affect this last
however long it's been has had on me. I feel
bruised down below, but in such a delicious
way. And the fear I felt at not knowing who
he was, the one thing that held me back from
truly enjoying it, has gone. My feet try to kick
my jeans off as a show of wanton availability,
no longer disgusted with the prospect. He
laughs quietly to himself, gazing at my
struggle as if it's amusing to him. Maybe it is,
but I want naked if I'm going to enjoy
whatever he's about to bring. I'd also like my
hands un-cuffed, so I can defend myself if

need be, but something tells me that's not going to happen.

"You'll be gentle, yes?" I stutter out, scanning his body.

He shakes his head and finishes his laughter with whatever thought he's had, muscles moving as he reaches for my legs. They're tugged towards him, jeans, boots and socks peeled off them slowly. "Not even if you beg, little Lilly," he says, throwing my clothes in the corner. "It will be painful and pitiless, and even when you think you're done, you'll scream for more of me."

Oh.

I don't know what to say to that, or think, but I still don't seem to be able to say the word 'no'. It just won't come out of me for any reason, regardless of his honesty. I flick my gaze away from him, trying to make sense of whatever my body is telling me to do. He's just a man, and there are plenty of others out there. Maybe not as attractive, and maybe not as able with their cocks as this one is but … I look at the handcuffs clipped around my wrist, for some reason interested in what they've done for me since I've been here. I enjoyed them, enjoyed him.

"You ready, Lilly?"

Yes. No.

I don't know.

The End

Anabella Roscoff

Hi, you've reached Anabella.

I'm not here.

I'm everywhere.

Don't forget to keep looking for more in the series. It will be ongoing, and full of everything naughty. Men, women. Men on men. Women on women. Several of each, and anything in between.

T's services spread extremely wide, and she always gives the client what they want regardless of the act required.

X

Printed in Great Britain
by Amazon